D0090445

Praise for *Hope Heals*

As I read this book, tears streamed from my eyes even as joy flooded my heart. Jay and Katherine are a raw yet refreshing testimony to the unshakable trustworthiness of God amidst the unimaginable trials of life. This book reminds all of us where hope can be found in a world where none of us know what the next day holds.

David Platt, author of the *New York Times* bestseller
Radical and president of the International Mission Board

Hope Heals is a beautiful, true story that illustrates the love and protection God has for us even in the darkest times of our lives. Katherine and Jay's dedication to each other and the Lord through their most devastating season is inspiring. This book will help your heart believe that He sees, He knows, He cares, and He is still working miracles today!

Lysa TerKeurst, *New York Times* bestselling author
and president of Proverbs 31 Ministries

Jay and Katherine Wolf have had our respect for years, but they have our hearts too. They'll soon have yours. *Hope Heals* isn't just a beautifully written book; it's a duet by two people who love Jesus and love each other. It's a book filled with a score of authentic high notes and painful low ones. This book isn't just a moving story; it's a song sung by two humble people and what they've learned about love when the cadence of their lives unexpectedly changed.

Bob and Maria Goff, balloon inflaters and author
of the *New York Times* bestseller *Love Does*

I stumbled upon Katherine's blog near the beginning of her recovery. The words of a sister fighting for her life captivated us all. Now years later, she is fighting for our lives—for us to live the fullest we can with all that we've been given. Do not miss this!

Jennie Allen, founder and visionary of IF:Gathering
and author of *Anything* and *Restless*

I know Jay and Katherine, and I welcome this book, not just as a stirring account of facing tragedy but as a beautiful story of a couple's relentless love—for God and for each other.

Philip Yancey, bestselling author of
What's So Amazing About Grace?

The book you hold in your hands is so powerful, for if awful things happen to you, you now have a guide . . . *Hope Heals* may well be your most treasured companion through great trial and pain . . . Do not assume you've "heard it all before." Theirs is a story so raw, visceral, and impossibly real that you can't help but identify.

Joni Eareckson Tada, bestselling author and founder
and CEO of Joni and Friends International

HOPE HEALS

HOPE HEALS

A TRUE STORY OF OVERWHELMING
LOSS AND AN OVERCOMING LOVE

WITHDRAWN

KATHERINE AND
JAY WOLF

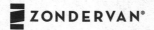 ZONDERVAN®

ZONDERVAN

Hope Heals
Copyright © 2016 by Katherine Wolf and Jay Wolf

Requests for information should be addressed to:
Zondervan, 3900 *Sparks Dr. SE, Grand Rapids, Michigan* 49546

ISBN 978-0-310-34739-2 (audio edition)

ISBN 978-0-310-34455-1 (ebook)

Library of Congress Cataloging-in-Publication Data

Names: Wolf, Katherine (Stroke victim) author.
Title: Hope heals : a true story of overwhelming loss and an overcoming love /
    Katherine and Jay Wolf.
Description: Grand Rapids : Zondervan, 2016.
Identifiers: LCCN 2015040951 | ISBN 9780310344544 (hardcover)
Subjects: LCSH: Wolf, Katherine (Stroke victim) | Cerebrovascular disease —
    Patients — Religious life.
Classification: LCC BV4910.6.C47 W65 2016 | DDC 248.8/6196810092 — dc23 LC
    record available at http://lccn.loc.gov/2015040951

All Scripture quotations, unless otherwise indicated, are taken from The Holy Bible,
New International Version®, NIV®. Copyright © 1973, 1978, 1984, 2011 by Biblica, Inc.®
Used by permission. All rights reserved worldwide. www.zondervan.com. The "NIV"
and "New International Version" are trademarks registered in the United States
Patent and Trademark Office by Biblica, Inc.®

Scripture quotations marked ESV are taken from The Holy Bible, English Standard
Version, copyright © 2001 by Crossway Bibles, a publishing ministry of Good News
Publishers. Used by permission. All rights reserved.

Any Internet addresses (websites, blogs, etc.) and telephone numbers in this book
are offered as a resource. They are not intended in any way to be or imply an
endorsement by Zondervan, nor does Zondervan vouch for the content of these
sites and numbers for the life of this book.

All rights reserved. No part of this publication may be reproduced, stored in a
retrieval system, or transmitted in any form or by any means—electronic, mechanical,
photocopy, recording, or any other—except for brief quotations in printed reviews,
without the prior permission of the publisher.

The names of all patients referred to in this book have been changed to protect their
privacy.

The author is represented by Alive Literary Agency, 7680 Goddard Street, Suite 200,
Colorado Springs, Colorado 80920, www.alivecommunications.com

Cover design: Micah Kandros
Cover photo: Emily Blake Photography
Photo insert: All photos courtesy of Jay Wolf III unless otherwise noted
Interior and photo insert design: Kait Lamphere

First Printing February 2016 / Printed in the United States of America

For James and John—
our daily reminders of healing and hope . . .

CONTENTS

FOREWORD
Before You Begin . . .

So there I was, sitting near the back of the room, listening to Jay and Katherine share their story. I wasn't expecting anything too new, given that I'm also in a wheelchair and Ken and I have a similar story. Plus, I have heard hundreds of couples talk about overcoming accidents and injuries. But this time, something felt different . . .

Part of it was the way they looked. Jay sat next to his wife, looking handsome, measured, and reasoned—the picture of thoughtful intelligence. On the other hand, Katherine spoke raspingly and loudly, and with sweeping gestures that made me fear she might fall out of her wheelchair. This was a fascinating couple to watch.

A brain stem stroke did all this? I wondered what they would say.

As Katherine shared about her first Thanksgiving out of the hospital, she described a poignant scene. The kitchen and family room were filled with people laughing, setting the table, and fixing dinner. Katherine sat in a corner, slumped in her wheelchair with her chin on her chest, staring at it all. She watched as her family fussed over her baby. Then, as if reliving the moment, she said, slowly and in a half whisper, "I looked at the scene before me and thought, *I don't think this world will work for me . . . It won't work.*"

This world won't work for me. How many times have I felt and said the same thing, given my own struggles with paralysis! Tears flooded my eyes, for here was a woman who had reached into the most tender part of my soul . . . and *touched* it. From then on, I was totally gripped by everything Katherine and Jay said from the platform. Although our situations were different, her story was my story. Her pain *fit*. She was able to look right through me and say, *I understand. I get it. I resonate with you.*

Isn't that what we all long for? Someone who will meld our heart with theirs? Someone who can validate our pain and assure us that if God got them through their mess, He'll get us through ours?

Besides, we all identify with pretty things that get broken. We sigh and feel sad when youth becomes horribly marred. We shake our heads and say, "What a shame!" if fate scrapes a beautiful smile from a fair innocent, leaving a damaged grin. We hate when that happens.

And *this* is why the book you hold in your hands is so powerful . . .

For if awful things *do* happen to you, you now have a guide. You have two seasoned warriors in Jay and Katherine who understand. You have two friends who can escort you through the grief and loss and out into the broad, spacious plain of peace and contentment. *Hope Heals* may well be your most treasured companion through great trial and pain. So please, don't plow through it too quickly. Read the Wolfs' story prayerfully and act on their counsel intentionally.

And I need to make a correction. Katherine's grin is far, *far* from damaged. Spend time with her and her husband, and you begin to understand what true beauty is all about. You understand how hard-fought-for their smiles really are, and that makes Katherine's grin the sweetest, most endearing expression you will *ever* see.

Does your world work for you? If not—or if it could be better—join me in the back of the room and listen to Jay and Katherine. Do not assume you've "heard it all before." Theirs is a story so raw, visceral, and impossibly real that you can't help but identify. You cannot help but resonate. So flip the page and get started. And as you journey beside Jay and Katherine, I pray that this hope—the kind that really heals—will touch the deepest part of *your* soul.

Joni Eareckson Tada,
Joni and Friends International Disability Center,
Agoura Hills, California,
Spring 2016

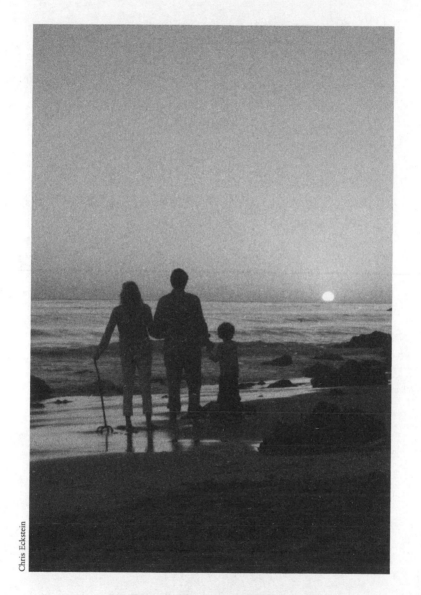

Chris Eckstein

PROLOGUE

Katherine

I imagine most of us have fairly straightforward pictures in our heads about what our lives will look like and who we will become. These pictures are mostly of wonderful things that happen at exactly the right time and make oh-so-much sense. When something happens that is not inside the four corners of that picture, we view it as a detour and hope to get back on track as quickly as possible.

So what happens when you take a detour and can't ever get back on that original path again?

I can tell you. The greatest detour anyone can take in life, I imagine, is a near-death experience.

Six months and five days after our beautiful, big-eyed baby James was born, I nearly died of a massive brain stem stroke. My family's journey over the past seven years has been arduous and so achingly slow that at times my husband and I have wondered how we could go on.

I've had eleven surgeries since my stroke. I've fought my way back to being able to do the most basic things again, and yet many disabilities remain. I can't do so many things I used to do and long to do now, and there is a profound sense of loss that lingers. Sometimes it feels like I'm an observer of my own life.

Surprisingly, on the far side of our tragedy, refined versions of our prior selves remain, ones that have walked with God through the fire but have not been consumed. Yet scars remain also, and it's been painful in ways I never thought possible. Having a small child makes it even more heartbreaking. Sometimes I feel so alone, even though I know that nothing is further from the truth. I *still* can't believe this happened to me, even though I've had years now to settle into my new reality.

Everyone asks if I've ever had a moment of total despair or hopelessness. The answer is yes and no. My feelings were hurt badly when this happened to me. At times I felt like God had made a mistake, and I struggled to make sense of all the pain. Several times I thought I should just end this. *I'm caught between life and death,* I reasoned. *This could not be what God planned for my life.* In those darkest moments, however, God spoke into that mess and revealed truth I already knew: He sees the entire picture, and HE DOES NOT MAKE MISTAKES. He knows this is part of the story He is writing for me, for my family, and for all of the creation He is making right. It is not a plan B, and I trust that.

Still, no amount of catharsis or perspective finding will change the fact that our situation is terribly sad and deeply broken. I can give God the glory, and it can still hurt. I used to cry myself to sleep every night. But I have learned, above all other lessons, that healing for each of us is spiritual. We will be fully restored in heaven, but we are actually healed on earth *right now.* My experience has caused me to redefine healing and to discover a hope that heals the most broken places: our souls.

What has happened to me is extreme; however, it is not that different from what everyone deals with. I am a sort of microcosm for what we all feel. I can barely walk, even with a cane, but who feels free even if they can? My face is paralyzed, but who feels beautiful even when they look normal? I have no coordination in my right hand, so I can't hold things, even my child, but who feels like a competent parent even if all their faculties are intact? For months I could not eat, and even today I have difficulty swallowing, but who feels fully satisfied even if they can enjoy every delectable treat they desire? I am tired almost all the time now, but who always feels energized to engage fully in their life? My voice is messed up, but who feels understood even if they can speak plainly? I have double vision, but who sees everything clearly even if they can see normally? My future is uncertain, but whose isn't?

So no matter the situation, universally people feel what I am living out. They don't feel free. They don't feel understood. They don't feel satisfied.

I believe that pain is pain, no matter what the form, but perspective is also perspective. Ultimately, ours is a story of a life overcome by hope. We are discovering joy even in the sadness and *choosing* contentment when it is very, very hard. For that, and for countless other blessings, I am so grateful to God. In some ways, Jay and I have been blessed to suffer greatly at such a young age because it informs the way we live the rest of our lives. We have learned that when everything else is gone, hope remains.

Perhaps some detours aren't detours at all. Perhaps they are actually *the* path. *The* picture. *The* plan. And, perhaps most unexpectedly, they can be perfect.

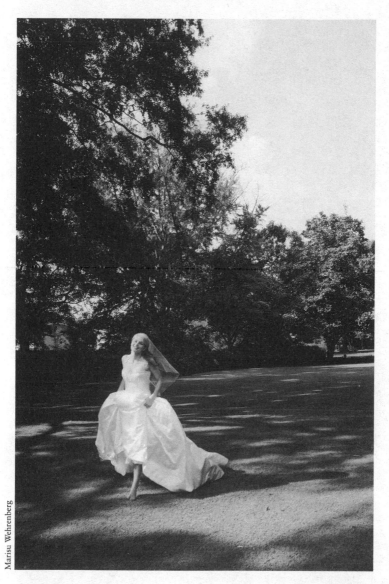

PART ONE

Marisu Wehrenberg

THE DREAM BROKEN

Katherine

I lay in bed at 4:00 a.m., unable to shake the sickening feeling. I had been up with James for a feeding an hour earlier and noticed then that something was off. I felt nauseous and spacy, and my head was pounding. My upper neck and shoulders were throbbing. Some of these feelings had been commonplace during my pregnancy, so I concluded that I needed to get my hands on a pregnancy test sometime the next day.

I tried to fall back to sleep despite the terrible nausea and an intense headache, knowing I had only a few hours until James would be awake and hungry again. The lack of sleep had deeply affected Jay and me in those first six months. Our marriage was in a tense season as we navigated life with a newborn. We still felt we were living in a bit of a dollhouse and should be able to turn off the crying switch on the baby doll's back. Instead, we lived in a sleepless haze and wondered when we'd ever feel "normal" again.

I finally drifted off, only to wake up a couple hours later, feeling like I could have slept for at least another eight. Still, I looked forward to a rare "free" morning of doing my son's endless laundry and cleaning up the apartment before heading out to the post office so I could get a bunch of thank-you notes in the mail. My grandmother and mother had instilled in me a thank-you-note-writing mentality, and as a true Southern belle, I could not enjoy the gift until the thank-you had been sent. At the three-week mark since Jay's and my annual joint birthday party, it was beyond time to mail the notes. I knew the consummate, etiquette-following lady never went to bed after receiving a gift until the note was written and ready for mailing the following morning. Yeah, right! Was this true once she had her babies? Did she somehow squeeze in note writing before 3:00 a.m. newborn feedings?!

After hitting the post office, we stopped at the grocery store, where I grabbed the ingredients for the meals I was planning to make for two families who had new babies. Back at home, with my baby boy settled in for his morning nap, I took the pregnancy test and was relieved to see the negative sign. *So what's wrong with me?* I wondered. *Food poisoning? Some weird virus? Lack of rest?*

I opened the First Baptist Montgomery cookbook to a lasagna recipe that was always a huge hit back home. For the next twenty minutes, I would be doubling ingredient quantities in my head and preparing sauce and browning ground beef. My nausea and headache were still there, but I had to push through those funky feelings and get the meals made. We had been the recipients of countless meals after James arrived, and I had seen how much it meant to us to not even have to think about preparing dinner. But now all I could think about was getting off my feet and closing my (now stinging) eyes. The room began spinning and suddenly felt way too bright. I needed soothing, low-lit surroundings. I made my way to the couch a few feet away, sure that if I just got off my feet for a moment I'd feel better. But as I sat down, it was as if all the blood in my body rushed into my head. I felt like I was choking and couldn't breathe.

"JAAAYY! COME IN HERE NOW! SOMETHING'S WRONG!"

I tried to stand, only to realize that my legs were numb. Everything in the room was now moving in a circle, but also coming in and out of focus and jumping from one place to another in my line of sight. Jay flew into the room and, frantic, screamed right in my face. *All this noise is going to wake up James*, I thought. *Jay's voice is so loud, and I need quiet.*

I tried to dismiss the thought that what was happening to me was anything serious. *What a drama queen I am,* I thought. *Why do I always make a scene? What will the neighbors think? This is so embarrassing.*

Then I heard Jay yelling into the phone.

Jay

After three long years, the end of my law school education was imminent. Though I was grateful to be done with the intense culture, testing, and expectations, Pepperdine had been our first home, and it would be very hard to leave.

On Mondays that last semester, I had about an hour between classes, right around noon. Leaving the mid-morning class, I realized I'd left some things at home that I needed to prepare for the final exam presentation I would be giving in my next class. I usually stayed on campus at lunchtime, but that day, April 21, 2008, I went back to our on-campus married housing apartment, brushing aside any shame over my procrastination in preparing for the final. We had a six-month-old baby—who could blame me for being spread a little thin? He was not on a schedule and didn't sleep through the night, so neither did we.

Katherine was cooking in the kitchen, and after giving her a quick kiss, I plopped down on an old chair squeezed into the corner of our bedroom. I began rifling through my scattered papers and typing words on the final slides for my presentation. Class would be starting within the hour, so I searched hastily for just the right pictures to add.

Suddenly, I heard Katherine's panicked call for me to "Come in here!!" She has always had a flair for the dramatic, but what could be important enough to possibly wake up James? I ran to the main room, where I found her seated on the couch in an unnatural slump. The TV was on, and she staggered across the living room floor toward the noise, mumbling that everything was too loud. The moment she touched the Off button, it was as if she turned herself off too. Her body fell hard onto the floor, sprawled, motionless.

The room closed in on me. I could almost hear the blood rushing through my ears and feel the adrenaline pump through my body. I sprang to her side, staring down at her normally animated frame, now seemingly lifeless. I cursed and yelled, not at her, but at my own realization that I was looking into the very face of death.

All I could see were her pupils. They were black, consuming almost every remnant of blue iris. Those blue eyes were one of the first things I saw whenever I saw Katherine. Her eyes could speak more expressively than most could with their words. But now it looked as though her light was being eclipsed by an unknown darkness. Her eyes were motionless, as if resigned to the fate of the expanding black hole of her pupils, the place into which everything would be sucked down forever.

Suddenly, Katherine gasped deeply and sat up, as if having been resuscitated on the beach after nearly drowning in the sea. No sooner did I, too, breathe a sigh of relief than she began to vomit violently. I propped her on some pillows and scrambled to find the phone. I had never dialed 9-1-1 before and was grateful it was easy to remember. Nonetheless, I fumbled and dialed 4-1-1 at least once before getting it right.

The operator had me elevate Katherine's legs on a chair and assured me that help was coming. It seemed that a veritable swarm of EMT workers poured through our front door almost as soon as I put down the phone. The sleepy beach town clearly had no other emergencies occurring then; their entire crew had come to this call. As I moved away from Katherine, stepping to the corner of the room to allow them to assess her, I was momentarily relieved but panicked, too, as though engaging medical professionals somehow made whatever was happening to Katherine more real, as if we could not go back to our ordinary day because of what I had set into motion by dialing those three numbers.

After quickly examining her, the head paramedic announced that they would be taking Katherine to the ER at UCLA Medical Center, Santa Monica, which was nearly half an hour down the Pacific Coast Highway, and that I should follow them in my car. They had already strapped her to a stretcher and were lifting the contraption up as one would do an ironing board, with the same screeching noise. Yet their fluidity and precision diffused some of the dizzying chaos that had exploded into our normally peaceful space.

Just beyond the stretcher on which Katherine lay, out the main window of our living room I saw the blue sliver of the Pacific Ocean. We loved saying our place had an ocean view, though it was mostly parking lot with a hint of ocean only if you looked at just the right angle on a cloudless day. Today was such a day, and I was standing at the right angle. That thin watercolor streak of ocean blue often faded right into the sky above so one couldn't tell where the ocean stopped and the sky began.

In a blink, I was transported back to another sliver of ocean blue, this one in Katherine's eyes. The blue irises were once again prominent, though visibly straining to overcome the blackness as her eyes darted around the room. A tear zigzagged down her cheek.

"Call Anna," she pleaded. "Get her to take care of James." Anna and Andy were some of our closest friends, and though pregnant with their first child, these not-yet-parents were the most knowledgeable on the subject of babies since nearly no one else in our friend group had had kids yet.

Katherine's words had an urgent, almost dying-wish quality to them, which terrified me. *What do you know that I don't know?* I thought, dread nearly capsizing me. "I love you," I told her. "Don't worry." I kissed her forehead, feigning confidence as my voice cracked. I gulped down the lump in my throat as the EMTs pushed the stretcher into the hallway in preparation for the trip down three flights of stairs. I could tell she wanted to turn her head or lift her hand to say good-bye, but her arms were strapped down tightly. The door to our apartment slammed shut so hard behind them that the welcome wreath attached to it crashed to the ground in a jarring clatter. Then all of a sudden, it was quiet again—until I heard the sound of my own wailing.

Katherine's emotional state was often contingent on mine, so I had maintained my composure until she was taken to the hospital. Now I could no longer hold in the wave of sobs. *What do I do now?* I raced to the bedroom to gather an overnight bag for her. Surely this insane detour would be over by tomorrow, and we would return home, grateful, maybe slightly embarrassed at all the fuss.

I threw into a bag Katherine's favorite pair of post-pregnancy lounge pants, which I hated. It made me smile to see them. I suppose she had earned the right to wear whatever pants she pleased. After grabbing her toothbrush, I couldn't think of anything else to pack. I proceeded to rouse James, who had impressively slept through the single most tumultuous twenty minutes of his life and ours. I grabbed his diaper bag and rushed downstairs to our car, half expecting to see Katherine being lifted gently into the ambulance, but she was long gone. I could barely make out the sound of a siren in the distance. I strapped James into his car seat and sped down the hill to leave campus.

I saw a law school friend walking to the class I was supposed to be attending. She waved, her smile quickly fading as I screeched to a halt next to her and tried to calmly yell that I would not be at class as Katherine was heading to the ER and could she please tell our professor. I floored it forward, bouncing on the campus speed bumps like a novice horseback rider. I groped around my pocket and the front seat for my cell phone but couldn't find it anywhere. I hit the steering wheel and screamed in frustration so violently that James began to cry, and I did too. I made a majorly illegal U-turn in the middle of the road, raced back up the hill, and parked on the curb with flashers blinking. Leaving James inside, I sprinted up the three flights of stairs, skidding into our apartment. I quickly found my phone, plugged in by my bedside next to the picture of Katherine running in her wedding dress—my favorite picture of her. I flew back to the car and drove off campus, calling Anna on the cell phone. She lived close to the hospital in Santa Monica, so I asked her to try to meet Katherine's ambulance there, as I would be lagging behind.

The mountains line one side of the Pacific Coast Highway, while the ocean nearly laps the other side. The road curves back and forth hypnotically, hugging the natural undulations of the mountain range. In the three years we had lived in Malibu, Katherine had put nearly 100,000 miles on our car, mostly traversing this same stretch of highway on her way to auditions and church and adventures with James. We always said if you had to have a commute, it might as well be this one. On this familiar route, I began to calm myself, remembering that every other time I had driven this road, Katherine was okay and alive and well, and this time would be no different.

No sooner had I soothed myself with such pat reassurances than I glimpsed James in the rearview mirror, visibly upset after being ripped away from his nap by a yelling, crazy person, and I remembered this drive was not a normal one. Suddenly, a deluge of horrific thoughts flooded me like a tsunami pent up behind a dam of sticks. *What if she dies? Today might be your day to see the worst life has to offer, to no longer be a casual observer of the pain but the recipient. What if she dies? Will you take*

James and move to Africa to serve the poor? Or will you go off the deep end and leave everything and everyone else, like Katherine left you? What if she dies? Today, it seemed that the target was on my back, and the arrow of brokenness quivered through the air to find its mark.

Like a plane coming out of a cloud bank, we suddenly arrived at the ER, and I tried to shake off the shroud of dark thoughts as I looked for parking. I pulled into the loading zone, not knowing where to go or what to do. And then I looked in the rearview mirror and saw one of the most horrifying sights of my life—our visibly pregnant friend Anna, her face ashen, brow furrowed, running toward our car. In that moment, I knew my deepest fear just might be coming true.

I began to sprint to the hospital entrance, my eyes searching for signage, my brain grappling with the affirmation of my great fears. This wasn't food poisoning or some post-pregnancy, freak blood sugar drop; no, this was something much bigger.

I ran up to the ER desk and manically asked the person seated behind it where I could find my wife. "What's her name," she asked calmly, in a way that reminded me this was *my* crisis, not the rest of the world's. "Her name's Katherine. Katherine Wolf. She just arrived by ambulance." The soft click of computer keys punctuated the silence, which lingered longer than my short-fused patience would allow. I left the desk and staggered around the hallway, just looking for Katherine instead. An older ER doctor apprehended me knowingly. "I'm looking for my wife," I nearly shouted. "The ambulance just brought her here. Something's very wrong." As I spoke the last words, I couldn't contain my whimpering sobs. The man, maybe of Eastern European descent, cupped my face in his hands and looked me right in the eyes in a way that denoted both authority and intimate commiseration. "Shhh, son, it's okay. She's here. She's here. We think she's had a stroke, and we will help her."

He quickly led me to the room where Katherine was surrounded by a new swarm of medical professionals. I called out to her, but her eyes were closed and she was motionless. A nurse was quickly cutting off her T-shirt, the one from our senior year in college when she had successfully chaired her sorority's recruitment campaign. She had chosen the color, a vibrant shade of Tiffany blue—her favorite. It was ripped off her and thrown to the floor in a shredded heap. Her bra was now exposed as they placed heart-monitoring pads on her chest. I lurched to pull the curtain or shut the door to give her privacy, but my new doctor friend held me back, shut the door to her room, and quietly and expertly guided me away to a private waiting room.

Within the hour, it became clear that UCLA, Santa Monica, a satellite hospital campus, wasn't as well equipped to help her as the main UCLA Medical Center in Westwood was, just a few miles down the road. There was a neurosurgeon on call there. I signed whatever release papers were handed to me without even looking at them and ran to my car with James and Anna in tow. I was not going to be so far behind the ambulance this time.

As I drove, I began to make phone calls to my parents and Katherine's. Hardly knowing what to say, I explained that she had been taken to the hospital and that she had had a stroke and that I would keep them posted. I raced to the next ER, where, plastered over the entrance, was a huge sign:

**#3 HOSPITAL IN THE COUNTRY,
BEST IN THE WEST.**

We were both twenty-six and healthy. We didn't even have a primary care doctor. I couldn't have told you where the nearest hospital was to our home in Malibu, much less which one was the best. And yet it was clear we had been brought to the right place.

I ran inside, scanning the room for another helpful, older-doctor figure. Instead, my gaze fell on some familiar, if out-of-place, faces. I blinked, confused. It was Monday midday; why were friends from our church in this waiting room? It quickly dawned on me that they were gathering there for us. This revelation both deeply comforted me and sickeningly proved the dark whisper in my head to be true: *This was a very serious matter.*

Dr. Nestor Gonzales, apparently one of the most highly respected neurosurgeons at UCLA Medical Center, approached me. His face was concerned, eyes sorrowful yet compassionate. "I will be treating your wife, Katherine," he said in a Spanish accent. "She has suffered a major neurovascular incident, and we will need to perform surgery immediately." In a gentle voice, he added, "I need you to know that there is a good chance she will not survive."

To experience such a reversal within the course of a few hours was more bewildering and disorienting than being flung upside down on a carnival ride. The world was still there, but this view of life was nearly unrecognizable. We had awakened to a normal day of law school presentations and baby diapers and preparing food and wondering where we would move after I graduated and if James would sleep through the night. Now the innocent myth of youthful immortality had burst like an iridescent bubble blown from a child's lips as Katherine lay dying.

I signed all the documents giving my consent for the surgery. I would later find out that shortly before our conversation, Dr. Gonzales had been wrestling with Katherine's case, weighing whether or not he should even attempt to do surgery, given the severity of her injury and the small likelihood of a positive outcome. He was even informed that I was an attorney. The circumstances, the liability, and the potentially huge expenditure of the hospital's resources weighed heavily against surgery. And yet he knew she had a six-month-old son. Though Katherine was already unconscious upon their meeting, he inexplicably felt she was entrusting her life into his hands, and despite the longer list of reasons not to operate, he felt undeniably compelled to give this young mother a chance to live.

As the doctor hurriedly left to prepare for surgery, I told him with surprising forthrightness, "I will—we all will—be praying for you." He nodded in grateful acceptance, as if he knew he would need all the prayers he could get.

Katherine's sister Amie had arrived, and we waited in the hallway for someone to direct us to Katherine's room. A resident matter-of-factly explained that we couldn't see her because they were drilling a hole in her skull right then in order to relieve some of the mounting pressure in her brain. I suddenly felt lightheaded, my body rocking back into the wall. I didn't normally do well with blood or hospitals, and the very thought of Katherine undergoing such a medieval-sounding procedure nearly undid me.

Then, out of the corner of my eye, I saw a patient being wheeled down the hallway on a bed. It was Katherine. I silently reached out my hand and touched her arm, unable to even stutter out, *Stop! This is my dying wife. I need to say good-bye.* Perhaps I didn't want to slow their journey to the OR, or maybe I thought this good-bye might well be the last of all our good-byes, the abstention from which might prevent its finality.

And then in my mind's eye flashed a different picture of Katherine—not the Katherine unconscious on the gurney, dressed in hospital whites, but the Katherine from the picture at my bedside, the Katherine smiling and running in her wedding dress, barefoot in the grass. That photo captures her perfectly, illuminated in a shaft of light, mid-stride, surrounded by the dappled shadows of an overhanging tree. I felt something shift inside me, like fresh life breathed into bursting lungs. I would refuse to let this tsunami tear me from Katherine. I would release myself into this unnatural life inversion, no longer fighting to be up-righted, no longer straining toward the life we knew that morning or the sinking thoughts that lured me deeper down and farther away. I would live upside down if it meant living upside down with her.

Across the crowded college cafeteria eight years before, I had seen Katherine for the first time. She was the most beautiful woman I had ever seen in real life, yet at the same time one of the most unexpectedly approachable. Perhaps it was her warm smile, or maybe it was her lunch tray overflowing with food. Either way, I was nearly speechless when she approached the round table I was seated at with a fraternity pledge brother of mine and asked to join us.

The cafeteria at Samford carried with it some of the archetypal high school seating code, and as it were, Katherine was pledging a sorority that was considered the sister to the fraternity I was pledging. I guess she was less approaching me as she was joining a "friendly" brotherly table, but nonetheless, she sat down. My friend had to go to class, so, like something out of a movie, I was left alone with this dream girl, who proceeded to chow down. She was easy to talk to and emboldened as only college freshmen can be, I engaged in some lively conversation with her until almost the entire room was empty. Seeing how much time had passed, she jumped up, needing to head back to her dorm. With uncharacteristic boldness, I asked her to go on a jog later to make up for the insane amount of calories we had both consumed. To my astonishment, she agreed!

Near dusk, we met in the well-traversed space between the freshman girl and guy dorms. In the warm evening air of early autumn, we briskly jogged the loop around campus. We chatted about our families and where we had come from. She also not so subtly mentioned her hometown boyfriend, who played football for the University of Georgia, and she kindly suggested I might like to go to a game sometime with her. It was a slight punch to the gut, but I was undeterred. Within the span of an afternoon, I was already falling for this lovely creature, her long, blonde ponytail whipping through the air as she excitedly bounced down the sidewalk, talking a mile a minute.

And then, in midsentence, her voice faltered, and I looked to my left in horror. I saw her long legs splayed out on the road as a result of falling off the sidewalk. No sooner did I yell and run to her aid than she sprang up from the road in a single, deer-like movement back onto the sidewalk. I stood slack-jawed for a moment, praying that our first "date" would not forever be marred by a broken bone or a bloodied knee. In what I would later find to be a classic "Katherine response," she yelled, "I'm fine! I've always been a klutz. Come on, catch up!" I knew at that moment that Katherine was a woman unlike any I had ever known.

Two months earlier, my parents and three younger sisters had driven me an hour and a half north of our home in Montgomery, Alabama, to Birmingham to move me into my college dorm. I had waited until the night before to pack virtually everything I owned into a dozen baskets, suitcases, and trash bags. We pulled onto the Rockwellian campus of Samford, which was abuzz with the frenetic energy of children metamorphosing into adults at that very moment. Perhaps for the first time, I felt like I just might find here something I'd been looking for for as long I could remember.

I have always wanted to do the right thing, if for no other reason than to give the appearance of one who always does the right thing. I am a firstborn, after all. I chaired the Honor Society and was awarded "Best All Around" (voted on by the teachers only) and didn't smoke or drink or date girls who did. Everything looked right on the outside, but internally I was deeply unsure of who I was and why I was.

I am the only boy, firstborn of four kids. My dad, a beloved pastor of a large church, and my mom, a hardworking stay-at-home, had both instilled in me the love of God and family. I think my heart formed in Washington, D.C., where I spent the bulk of my childhood, but my head formed in the Deep South, where I spent my youth. Those places shaped me profoundly by their contrasts, but in terms of finding myself, those juxtaposing experiences left me feeling a bit like a stranger in my own home.

Growing up in the church added to this conflict of self. I saw a real and beautiful, if messy, behind-the-curtain picture of Christian community, particularly at home, and it changed me in the best way. I knew God and loved God from an early age. But the Christian culture of the Bible Belt, one that was at times indistinguishable from the broader culture, was confusing.

Pulling up to the freshman dorm at Samford, something about the place caused me to think I might find the answers I was looking for. Maybe it was the newness, a different crowd of people, the separation from home, the chance to start over. As the student greeters helped me and my family to unload an ungodly amount of my junk from our van, I wondered if I'd feel like that same kid with a Virginia accent shut out of the Southern middle school sleepover. Yet, over the next few days, even hours, it became apparent that this place would be a new home. I quickly began to shed parts of my old persona—the insecurities and fears—and met new people from all over, people who thought I was interesting and dateable and funny. I was almost giddy with a sense of finally belonging.

I didn't have a clue what I wanted to major in or what I wanted to do with my life. I didn't have a clue what all was in store for me. But after that first run with Katherine, I somehow knew she would be a part of it. I had no idea of the issues in her brain that explained some of her charming klutziness, but I did have an uncanny sense of certainty that I wanted to love and care for this exquisite, spastic, vibrant girl. On that October day, I could never have imagined where that would lead us.

Katherine

To this day, I can't put my finger on exactly what drew me to Jay. He was completely unlike any guy I had ever dated. Perhaps that was what interested me all along.

I had had two serious boyfriends in high school. Both of them were major athletes, superpopular, life-of-the-party types. Both would go on to play college-level sports.

In contrast, Jay was unassuming, creative, scholarly yet wildly funny too, and deeply humble.

I loved that Jay was thoughtful about his faith, even while wrestling with it. I saw that he yearned to make his relationship with God personal rather than sliding into a more comfortable, cultural faith or one that simply rode the coattails of his pastor-father's legacy. He intrigued me, but I had no romantic interest in him whatsoever. I think, initially, he was the brother I'd never had.

Growing up, I attended an elite college prep school in Athens, Georgia, for fourteen years. The prevailing expectation was that graduating seniors would either enroll in the beloved state school located in our hometown or be accepted to a prestigious institution for higher learning that boasted strong name recognition and fabulous academics. True to form, I was on my way to the South's closest interpretation of an Ivy League school in the spring of my senior year. My parents' minds were set. My teachers' minds were set. And I thought my mind was set too.

As college plans were solidifying, I happened to go to a summer camp reunion in Birmingham, Alabama. In need of a place to stay during the reunion, I called up a sweet friend from Athens who was attending Samford University, a small, private Christian liberal arts school in Alabama. I'd never even heard of the place. I figured that while I was in town I would visit her, check out her dorm, eat in a real college cafeteria (honestly, I was most excited about that part!), and meet her new friends. Although we had not attended the same high school, I considered my friend a role model. I loved this beautiful, fabulous woman of God, who would later become my big sister in our sorority and a bridesmaid at my wedding.

I fell in love with the gorgeous campus, the incredible people, and Samford's dedication to supporting my faith. Former plans forgotten, I decided I simply *had* to go there! The previous fall, I had won the award for "Best Actress in the State of Georgia" at a one-act play competition, which prompted my desire to pursue theatre in college. So, naturally, by the time my mom picked me up in Birmingham at the end of my summer camp weekend, I had already arranged for us to meet with the head of Samford's theatre department. I auditioned for him that very day and was subsequently offered a theatre scholarship for the fall. Now I *really* had to go to this college.

My parents had never heard of Samford, either. However, in their great wisdom, they trusted God's clear call on this place for their high-achieving, firstborn child. My parents never could have known why God navigated me away from my perfect plan and directly to Samford's gates. But, you see, He knew why. He knew Katherine Arnold had to get to Samford University to meet Jay Wolf and to find the place where their love story would begin.

We became best friends during our first semester in college. It was hard to find one of us without the other. I had a wonderful feeling of total safety with Jay. He was deeply kind and compassionate and had this "ability to listen" thing that was electrifying. I could talk to him for ten hours straight (seriously) and still have so much to say. While my walk with Jesus never felt very outstanding, I had always wanted Him and all of His amazing attributes in my life. Jay embodied many of these characteristics. There was a quality about him that I had never seen in a man before. He was so strong and wise, and yet unpretentious at the same time. Having three younger sisters, he had learned how to treat a female and deeply respect her. He was totally honoring of me in every way possible. Though he was on a journey of figuring out who he was—and making some mistakes along the way—I had never known a male to be so kind in my entire life.

During that time, I was dating a high school boyfriend who would become the all-time leading scorer on the Georgia football team. My entire life and identity were wrapped up in this hometown hero, and I would drive home almost every weekend for games. In November of our freshman year, our big sorority formal fell on the same day as one of the biggest college football games of the year, so my boyfriend was unable to attend. I needed a safe date. After much deliberation, Jay seemed the obvious choice. Even though I would never want any relationship with him beyond the sweet brother-sister thing for which we had become infamous on campus, I knew he was an absolute blast at any party that involved dancing. He has tremendous rhythm and loves to cut a rug, and I thought I could hide my superawkward tall-girl dance moves while laughing out loud the entire night.

And laugh we did! We danced right in front of the live band for more than three hours straight, with laugh-until-you-almost-wet-your-pants hoots and hollers. It was such a blast, surprisingly so—but at the same time, maybe not so surprising. As the evening ended, I couldn't shake this weird feeling. *Why was I so comfortable around Jay? We could never date or anything like that. Could we? This guy is like the brother I never had, so why am I starting to be so drawn to him as more than that?*

He had not told me that night, but I later learned that Jay had jeopardized his presidential scholarship by skipping a mandatory retreat to attend the formal with me. I felt horrified on one hand (thankfully, he got to keep the scholarship), but on the other hand, I felt valued and special. He was willing to take a risk and give up something really important, not out of obligation, but because he wanted to be with me. I had never met a man like this, and I knew then that I wanted to be with him too.

Jay

I managed to slowly but surely work my way into Katherine's affections, and over the course of becoming close friends, dating, breaking up, dating, breaking up, Katherine and I had history, but did we have a future? By the time we were seniors, I felt more confident in myself than I ever had in my life, more ready for the next season, and Katherine did too. The typical firstborn, Bible Belt responses of either rebellion or judgment (personified in myself and Katherine, respectively) had now given way to self-assuredness, a deep desire for authenticity, and a healthy dose of humility. We had lived in a place where the consequences were not totally real, and yet it naturally set the stage for us to take what we had learned and make the leap together into the real world.

As we approached the last semester of our college career, the question of the final status of our relationship loomed as well. After much thought and deliberation, Katherine felt drawn to pursue a career in the entertainment industry after college. She had become somewhat of a big fish in a small pond in the Southeast world of commercial print modeling, so she and a friend had been scheming a cross-country move to Los Angeles, where she could give it a shot in the big pond.

It was clear we were at a crossroads. It wasn't that I felt I needed to protect Katherine or jealously manage her journey in a city like LA; it was more that I didn't want to miss out on any life with her. I had dreams for my own future, but more than a concretized career path, I had dreams of spending my life with someone who got me, who challenged me to grow, and who loved me in spite of it all. Someone like Katherine.

But before this future could begin, I needed to ask her an important question.

I'm a creative at heart, so I knew I wanted our engagement to be a meaningful representation of our separate stories joining into one. Katherine, while sentimental to a degree, hates surprises and would have probably been fine with me popping the question in our beloved cafeteria between dessert courses. Instead, I schemed for months, gathering and framing dozens of pictures that charted both our histories, culminating with a picture of the inside of her hometown church, where I hoped we would be married. I even memorized a song that was sung at the end of every summer at the camp she had attended as a camper and counselor (the same camp reunion that spurred her to go to Samford). This song was a kind of calling to a close on a chapter of childhood and an invitation to a new chapter of life with me. Plus, I knew that Katherine so loved when I sang to her that she would likely do whatever I asked afterward.

On February 2, 2004, we drove down to my hometown—Montgomery, Alabama—on the pretext of visiting family. A proposal in my home church seemed just right, as it had not only been an integral part of my life for the many years my dad had served there, but Katherine had also been lovingly embraced by the church as one of its own. As I drove, Katherine fell asleep in the car, unknowingly peaceful in comparison to my hidden anxiety. I remember looking at her sleeping, my mind tumbling with nerves and awe that this complicated and amazing woman's life had collided with mine. God had brought us so far since the first day we met three and a half years before. I slyly texted my family that we were close to the church, where they had already scattered candles and flowers around the sanctuary and placed the framed pictures.

As we walked up the outer stairs to the sanctuary under some flimsy guise I had quickly constructed, it became very clear to her that something else was going on, particularly as she glimpsed candlelight flickering inside. Her eyes began to grow larger and glisten with tears of surprised understanding as a smile bloomed on her face. We entered, and I walked her down the middle aisle of the church that had been home for most of my life. With its red-tiled roof and marbled facade modeled after the Duomo in Florence, Italy, its monumental Tiffany stained glass angels keeping silent vigil, it may have been the last thing one would expect to see in that once-forsaken downtown, but somehow it had a place, and it wasn't going anywhere. Now, neither were we.

I don't remember much from the few minutes that followed, save for the memories reignited after the fact by the shaky video footage covertly taken by my dad from the back of the church. I sang the camp song to Katherine as I led her to the altar. I gave her a Bible with her would-be married name— "Katherine Wolf"—engraved in gold into its black leather. I narrated the disparate stories of our lives through the dozens of framed pictures, the moments that led us to the intersections that had led us to that very moment on the altar and would (hopefully) lead us, in the not-too-distant future, to her hometown church sanctuary for our wedding. I don't even remember asking her the question, but I remember shouting, "She said YES!" into the seemingly empty sanctuary, as my parents and sisters ran out from behind columns and pews in celebration. Our tight-knit family of six would expand to bring in this very different but already loved new member. They were overjoyed, and so were we.

As Katherine excitedly recounted the event to her parents on her cell phone, I quickly ascertained that the song I sang to her was not the iconic final song from her camp days; in fact, she didn't know the song and probably wondered why in the world I had sung it to her. I had been misinformed; yet rather than feeling deflated at my falling short of long-planned-for perfection, I was inflated as Katherine breathlessly described the moment as if it was the most perfect song that could have ever been chosen. The words are inspired by the blessing from Numbers 6: "The LORD bless you and keep you; the LORD make his face shine on you and be gracious to you; the LORD turn his face toward you and give you peace." The words are sung to the tune of "Edelweiss" from *The Sound of Music,* Katherine's absolute favorite childhood movie, watched on repeat during idyllic weekend stays with her much-adored grandparents.

I couldn't have planned it better if I had tried. It was an early foretaste of who Katherine would be to me—an encourager of my gifts, a fosterer of my best, albeit imperfect, efforts. She saw my heart, even when I had a hard time seeing it myself.

Katherine

Nine months of engagement *seemed* long enough to prepare for our nuptials. Once we set the wedding date, however, life seemed to speed up, and we couldn't slow it down. My initial ideas about an intimate wedding for our "closest friends and family" quickly succumbed to pressure to hold a blow-out gala in all its Southern-fried goodness. My family had lived in my small hometown for more than fifty years, and Jay and I were some of the first of our friends to marry, so our wedding was sure to be an event for the whole community. At more than six hundred guests, we probably should have just put ads in the paper: "Come one, come all!" Until our funerals, it's unlikely that so many people we love will be in the same room at the same time. But we both knew this wedding was not just about us. Printed in our wedding program was Psalm 115:1: "Not to us, LORD, not to us but to your name be the glory, because of your love and faithfulness." This was a glorious day to honor our Lord for our lives and point our friends and family to the true Giver of all good gifts.

November in Northeast Georgia is stunning. Though there was a chill in the air, it was still warm enough to be outside and enjoy the gorgeous colors of all the falling leaves. Surrounded by our beloved families and friends (and quite possibly a few strangers!), we entered that same sanctuary where my parents were married almost three decades before. Jay's dad officiated at the ceremony and spoke of the need to "build our house on the rock" and lay a foundation that would endure—because the storms of life come to everyone. We think the Lord knew we needed to have that truth planted deep in our souls. At twenty-two, we were both bright-eyed in love and perhaps a little naive as to what we were promising before God and those witnesses. Yet we gave each other heartfelt assurances of our devotion, words of hope and commitment that would be tested much sooner than we could have ever imagined.

After the noonday ceremony, we celebrated with a bright and festive reception, overflowing with my favorite Southern brunch foods like sweet potato biscuits and shrimp and grits, a towering white wedding cake and scrumptious chocolate and peanut butter groom's cake. The only minor tragedy of the day is that we didn't get to eat a bite of wedding food during our entire reception! We had spent many months adjusting and tweaking our menu, but the buffet style combined with the crowd would prevent us from getting to the good eats! (It worked out fine—our wedding planner made us a picnic feast we enjoyed afterward.)

Our first dance was to "Son of a Preacher Man," with lyrics personalized just for us. I didn't begin to grasp at the time how important those words would become in our story. Being a preacher's son's wife meant I had a husband who had grown up learning how to love people well. As an added bonus, it also meant we had a massive, built-in support system from the beginning. We were woven into a vital Christian community, and this would prove to be an immense gift. I loved watching our separate worlds collide on the dance floor as kids from Jay's church danced with kids from my neighborhood and Jay's grandmother followed my uncle in a spontaneous conga line. It was a precious slice of heaven.

Perhaps the most meaningful touch to our day was the framed black-and-white photographs of our mothers and grandmothers on their wedding days. We placed them in the entrance to the reception hall. While each marriage has known struggle and hardship through the years, our parents and all four sets of grandparents began their love story at a wedding while they were also quite young (early twenties) and continued it until death (or are still writing it—both sets of our parents have been married for more than thirty years). Because of that legacy of commitment, for better or worse, we knew that marriage was for life. And that is what we wanted.

Following all the festivities, we crossed the country and the Pacific to Hawaii for our first big "adult" vacation, though we technically weren't even old enough to rent a car.

After years of dating and questions about our future relationship and after months of stressful planning for the big wedding day, there was such a sense of release in being officially married and just being together at last. Our adventure as husband and wife had begun, and it was going to be an adventure beyond anything we could imagine.

Jay

Months before the wedding, we had taken a reconnaissance trip to Los Angeles with Katherine's folks. Katherine's agent in Birmingham had arranged a meeting with a top commercial and print modeling agency in Beverly Hills, and after meeting and chatting, they invited her to go on her first "casting" before returning home. She booked that job and subsequently signed with the agency. The start of her career was in the bag before we'd even moved and while we were in the thick of wedding planning.

I didn't know what I wanted to do after graduating from college with a double major in communication studies and Spanish and a minor in political science, nor did I know yet what my life's passion was. Thankfully, I had the voices of my parents and Katherine to help me uncover what was deep inside. Given my natural skills in writing and argument, pursuing a legal career began to emerge as a natural fit.

While in Los Angeles, we visited some of the law schools in the area. The campus of Pepperdine University in Malibu ascended from the Pacific Ocean, dotting a hillside like beautiful white and terra-cotta remnants from the high tide. It was overwhelmingly clear that this place could be an amazing home in which to live out our first years of marriage. We could envision our lives there, but one little issue remained: I needed to get in!

Back in Alabama, Katherine spoke at a women's event for older supporters and alumnae of our college and met a woman whose retired husband was once a dean at Pepperdine and was best friends with the law school's famous dean emeritus. She graciously connected us with this man, Dr. Ron Phillips, who is credited with starting and growing Pepperdine's law school as its longtime leader. On a second reconnaissance trip to LA, we met with Dr. Phillips, a man who is both erudite and grandfatherly. I shared with him my journey and my desires for our future. I even felt led to disclose a particularly low point in my college experience, a legal indiscretion that forced me to question the direction my future was heading, which ultimately changed the course of my life. In typical California fashion, he was gracious and unruffled, even pleasantly surprised at my candor, given that this was an interview in the legal field, not one known for its vulnerability and forthrightness.

I submitted the endless enrollment paperwork and studied for the dreaded LSAT, making a decent enough score to not be shamed in my application. I have never been an overly confident person, certainly not in areas outside my expertise or life experience, but I had a sense of peace about my future with Pepperdine.

After our wedding and honeymoon, we spent our first holidays together, expertly portioning ourselves out between our two families. As January 2005 arrived, we made the final preparations to pack up our lives to move twenty-five hundred miles away from everyone and everything we knew. Somewhere between Austin and El Paso, my mom called, excited to report that the law school acceptance letter had arrived in the mail. I was accepted into the school as one of about 250 first-year students out of thousands of applicants. I breathed a huge sigh of relief as we continued the journey to that glorious life by the sea. We were tingling with excitement at the chance to do something new, something that felt important somehow. The whole thing seemed beyond our comfort level and abilities, but the confidence of youth and two not-yet-fully-formed brains help in doing things that one would not dare consider a decade later.

We had a fun, fairly uneventful road trip, plodding our way across stretches of road we had never seen before, talking for hours about what we hoped lay ahead for us. As we were nearing the final stretch—literally the last few miles before our exit—a strange anxiety hit us both. Our printed-out directions indicated our new home was close, yet the surrounding big-city squalor looked anything but homey. I got off the 101 freeway exit to Santa Monica Boulevard. I knew there had been a song about this place, one with a sweet tune, one that sticks in your head for way too long; maybe it would be the new soundtrack to our new life.

I expectantly turned onto this famous thoroughfare but slammed on the brakes in horror to avoid a veritable conga line of people in the middle of the road. What lay ahead on Santa Monica Boulevard looked more like a developing country's bustling central marketplace than a convertible driver's golden path to a nearby beach pier's Ferris wheel. Katherine began to cry. I assured her that our actual street was surely miles away from this mob-sized crowd that was not heeding the crosswalk signs. A 97 Cents Store loomed large just ahead, and a few blocks beyond, I could just make out the street sign with the name of our new street. I considered driving past it and making a mile-long block to circle back around to it, but I was pretty sure I might get lost and possibly end up back on the not-so-beachy part of Santa Monica Boulevard. I swung the car onto our new street, feigning my own confidence while secretly wanting to throw up. *What will my in-laws think when they see where I've taken their daughter?*

We had found this apartment in an online classified ad, and we had excitedly agreed to rent it, sight unseen, with a zeal that only bright-eyed twenty-two-year-olds could muster. It was roughly three times the amount we had paid for our college apartments, but we were fairly confident we had snatched up a gem, assuming anything with the word *Hollywood* attached to it would have a certain innate shimmer. Turns out, it did have a certain shimmer, but I think it was urine. At least it was an actual apartment building and not some sort of scam to harvest our organs on the black market. To be fair, the online pictures were not that far from the reality, and the place did have a certain charm to it. From our doorstep, framed by the palm trees lining our street, we could even see the Hollywood sign on the distant hill.

Nonetheless, as the sun began to set on our first day in this new town—on our first day of adulthood, really—we felt a deep sense of needing to get behind a locked door. We began unloading our monogrammed toile bedspread and wedding china and various lamp shades from our packed-to-overflowing car. We then rapidly threw everything else inside the apartment, likely breaking a few items that had survived the trip, for fear that our car might be broken into if we left so much as a wedding tchotchke inside. We locked the door behind us, heaving a tentative sigh of relief. Like it or not, we were home.

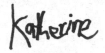

Before even moving to LA, the question posed at our wedding echoed in our heads: "What will be your foundation?" We were drawn to the adventure of a new place, the opportunity to engage new people and a new culture, and the possibility of realizing some long-held dreams, but we knew no one who lived in LA. We were each other's sole support system. We knew we would need something besides just one another to build a strong faith in our adult life.

Though young and headstrong and ready for independence, we knew that seeking out a church community would be integral to finding our way in this new life.

Interestingly, as we gathered LA-area church recommendations prior to moving, Bel Air Presbyterian Church kept coming up: "Oh, my nephew attends this great church," or "I went to school with a guy who was on staff there." We wrote out our church visiting list and put "Bel Air Pres" at the top.

On our first Sunday in town, we nervously crisscrossed Mulholland Drive, a winding road that snakes its way across the Santa Monica mountain range, the highest point in LA. Bel Air Presbyterian Church sits atop a spectacular overlook, with a valley full of homes and souls below it as far as the eye could see. We had never been to a church like this one.

That day, we also found the closest thing we could to a "Sunday school" class in a group of couples who gathered together between the morning services. What a revelation to engage a community that was in our same stage of life! We were elated to have found this potential new church home in such a sprawlingly anonymous city on our first Sunday. Later that afternoon, we returned to our apartment to find the Young Marrieds group leader had already left us a message, thanking us for coming. At that moment, we both knew our church shopping had ended before it even began.

Within nine months of arriving to LA, we moved from our first home in Hollywood to the married housing dorms on Pepperdine's campus. This new location in Malibu put us nearly an hour away from our new church home, but we felt called to continue engaging this exciting new community. Before too long, we did the good Southern volunteer thing and agreed to lead the Young Marrieds group at church. We were twenty-four years old and had been married about two years. Though we had no business leading a group of couples, many of whom had been married longer than we had, God was preparing us for something. We pored over marriage books and studied the Bible as we counseled friends who had marriage problems, and we cultivated a vibrant community of couples seeking to look like Jesus in a city that celebrates anything but that.

We connected to a small group, which met during the week and provided a more intimate experience. That group became like family. In LA, as in most big cities where the inhabitants are largely transplants, a strange thing happens within the context of community. It's as if you are watching the story of friendship unfold in fast-forward. The intensity of the need to not be alone can pull you together with a surprising force. Within weeks and months, you are no longer just new friends; you are doing life together. Beautiful and complicated, you become this kind of family that takes care of their own. We had found our people, our tribe.

Those first years of living in LA in this Christian community felt reminiscent of the euphoria of our freshman year of college, except it was even better because we were making new friends with our *best* friend by our side. That same college-era desire to belong was deepened and now attached to a sense of precise purpose. At the intersection of community and calling lies the body of Christ. Though we had known this truth for most of our lives, those first years in LA were like seeing it anew, because this time we chose it and gave it everything we had, not because we had to but because we wanted to. We belonged to it, and it was ours.

While my legal education entered its unglamorous second year, Katherine's career had been progressing in the surprisingly unglamorous world of commercial modeling and acting auditions. The shiny facade of the entertainment industry was beginning to slip, revealing more of its true form, and yet for this season, her work helped us pay the bills and was hopefully paving the way for bigger and better opportunities.

Katherine had a modeling gig in Palm Springs, a few hours outside of LA, so I drove her there to enjoy the free hotel offered by the job. After the job, we found a hole-in-the-wall Mexican restaurant—our favorite kind—and had a blast, loud-laughing and talking about the future over guacamole and enchiladas. That night, Katherine woke up with sharp stomach pains, far worse than the normal repercussions of said Mexican fare, so bad, in fact, that I toyed with taking her to the ER. They dissipated soon enough and were quickly forgotten. On the return trip home, we bought a bag of fresh grapefruit, the scent of which provoked Katherine to an unexpected revulsion so great that she violently flung them to the backseat of the car.

A few days later, we got together with some friends, who began sharing the wife's new venture, a Scripture-based meditation for a no-fear birthing experience. This was completely out of our normal headspace, as we had decided, as recently as our Palm Springs Mexican fiesta, that we would plan to have our first child around the age of thirty. This would give us just enough time to establish our careers, so Katherine might then take early motherhood retirement after publicly thanking God for her first Academy Award, and I would effortlessly manage my shockingly lucrative legal real estate career while simultaneously being lauded as Dad/Husband of the Year. We were twenty-four years old at the time.

Katherine always asks a lot of questions (apparently she has since the moment she could talk!), but this time her line of questions to our friend was strangely specific: "What does it feel like when you are newly pregnant, just curious . . . Would one feel sensitive in any way?" Our knowledgeable friend rattled off some early symptoms of pregnancy, including nausea, intensified sense of smell, tenderness in the breasts, and emotional sensitivity.

On our way home, Katherine made a rather flustered stop at the drugstore, and upon returning to our married housing dorm, she diverted herself to our bathroom as I went to a pile of schoolbooks. Within a few minutes, I heard, "JAY! Come here,

NOOOOW!" I ran to the bathroom to find Katherine leaning over the double sink vanity, looking in the mirror, breathing heavily, her mouth the definition of slack-jawed. It was like a scene from a movie or, at the very least, one of her acting classes. I almost laughed and rolled my eyes, until I noticed what was clutched in her hand—a pregnancy test. "What? Oh my . . . How?" I choked out. "You know HOW!" she growled back. "My mom always told me the women in my family are very fertile!"

After a few moments, the sense of riding a bike into a brick wall dissipated slightly, and we stared at each other and began to laugh uncontrollably. *How stupid did we have to be to not know how to use birth control?* "I think we need a second opinion," I stated reassuringly. No need to freak out. Perhaps there was some kind of fluke on the home pregnancy test.

Despite the ritzy connotation of Malibu, it's really just a sleepy beach town, which at the time had only one urgent care center. We rushed there as if a limb needed to be reattached and were promptly (and quite happily) given a $200 pee-in-this-cup test. The doctor came in the room and matter-of-factly confirmed, "Oh, yeah, you're pregnant, all right." But what he said next changed everything for us. "You know you don't have to keep it. You have options," he said, all grandfatherly, but not at all. In that moment, our incredulous, dumbfounded processing of this unexpected pregnancy turned into a visceral, steely resolve. Getting pregnant at twenty-four was not at all what we pictured for the first years of our marriage, but in that moment, a switch flipped in our minds, in our plans, in our future. This was *our baby*, just arriving six years earlier than we had thought. There was no other option, and we didn't want any other option.

We quickly left that place with a mix of inexplicable disgust and feverish purpose and proceeded to what was potentially the only worse place to go than that urgent care center—a

Babies"R"Us. Somehow we thought it might have some answers, some direction. Maybe deep down we knew we would find kindred spirits there who were also grappling their way through this greatest of life transformations. Suffice it to say, our senses were so overwhelmed (Katherine's were a little on edge already, as previously noted) that we left within a few minutes of arrival, and we haven't returned to one since!

The roller coaster of emotions we had been riding in that short span of time left us exhausted, so much so that we finally just crashed on the bed together, staring at the ceiling, utterly spent but now calm, enfolded in a surprising sense of peace. This was not the plan, but it was our plan now. With the same grit that led us to a new life far from home, we would figure out how to make our way in this world that looked totally different to us now.

Katherine

There was a time when I didn't understand why I had a baby at twenty-five. When I got pregnant, I worried about what it would mean for my career and my future. As an accomplished, type-A woman, I wondered if this baby would throw all my plans for a loop. As it turned out, he saved my life.

My pregnancy was perfectly healthy from beginning to end. Those forty weeks (and four days) before James made his appearance were fairly noneventful. I did have terrible morning sickness and extreme fatigue, but nothing that indicated what was actually happening inside my body.

James Thompson Wolf, our unexpected miracle, came into the world on October 16, 2007. Jay was a saint throughout the entire birthing experience. I think he rubbed my feet for eight of the ten hours of labor (the other two hours I would not permit any touching or any movement). His bedside manner was sooth-ing and deeply kind. I felt safe with him at the helm.

My mom and sister were also there. The women of the Arnold family do not know calm, but I do love them for it—"never boring," as my dad says! We are all drama queens and alarmists. My mom crawled into my hospital bed, braided my hair, and whispered the benefits of an epidural, despite my desire to not have one. She did the signature "Arnold scream" a few times during my labor, but she bravely held one leg while Jay held the other during the pushing. My sister Amie, who is only twenty-three months younger than me, went on a quick errand to fetch a phone charger two blocks away and came back three hours later with a bag full of burritos. She pushed her way to the foot of my bed (despite Jay's efforts to manhandle her out) and sobbed in horror as she witnessed James's arrival. She later hysterically cried because James had a "conehead," which she was sure would stay that way forever.

I had been laboring for ten hours with James in an extremely painful "sunny-side up" position, which caused masses of blood vessels to burst in my eyes from the intense strain. But he was well worth the wait. When he was finally placed on my chest, I cried with joy, while he just cried. We fell immediately in love with this precious little person who got to come home and live at our house *permanently*. My biggest decision after a healthy delivery was whether to have apple or cranberry juice in the recovery room. If only I had fully appreciated the simplicity of the kind of decisions I was called to make at that innocent time in my life.

Aside from sleep deprivation, the first six months with our baby were joyous and carefree for me. I was enjoying explor-ing new motherhood with my little buddy in tow. James began modeling with me, and we were booked on mother-son mode-ling jobs throughout his early life. We would drive up and down the Pacific Coast Highway for daily adventures and playdates in

Los Angeles. Jay was in his final year of law school at Pepperdine while adjusting to fatherhood. We were among the first of our friends to have a baby, and James became the mascot for our large group of twentysomething friends. He was everybody's baby. We liked it that way. James had many "aunts and uncles," which was all part of God's perfect plan. He was a communal baby all along. He had a village behind him.

James was too young to know that the fate of his mother was in his tiny hands, but in hindsight, it makes perfect sense. Had my son not been born "too early," he would not have been born at all, because six months and five days later, I would not have been able to deliver a baby. James and I would not have been given the chance to know each other in this life as mother and child.

While conceiving James was a total surprise to Jay and me, now I know that one reason he came into the world when he did was to give me a reason to fight for my life . . .

Jay

After Katherine was whisked off to surgery at UCLA, I was directed to a yellow line that would lead me from the ER waiting room to the OR waiting room. It wasn't exactly a yellow brick road, but a harrowing journey was clearly beginning. As I walked the line, a shift occurred, and my perspective became detached, like watching a film of myself methodically walking a yellow tightrope, as if with the slightest misstep all would be lost. Behind me trailed a quiet collection of the familiar faces of those friends who had dropped whatever they were doing in the middle of their Monday afternoons and had come to be with me. They were part ragtag army, part funeral processional. In that surreal, disembodied dirge, there was a surprising sense of integration, like all these disparate pieces and people were somehow coming together.

As we flooded out of the elevator into our destination, a rising sense of communal purpose came with us. The self-preserving mechanisms of shock and grief gave way to love. Though I had been around church people my entire life, something altogether unique began happening in and among us, something altogether spiritual. In such times of shock, often the most natural response is, "God, where are You?" I suppose in that moment, I realized that when we most need our intangible God to be made tangible, we need look no further than His people to make Him manifest.

Not long after we had settled into the new waiting room, I was called to collect Katherine's personal belongings from the pre-op suite. A surgical assistant handed me a bag of Katherine's clothes and took special care to give me a little baggy with Katherine's wedding rings in it. "They had to cut the wedding band off because her finger was too swollen to remove it." I gasped. Somehow the sight of those two pieces of broken metal felt like a punch in the gut. I remembered my dad's words at our wedding before we exchanged our rings. "These look like pretty great rings," he said. "They're made of some of the strongest, most valuable metals around. Each time the sun glints off them or you feel them twist on your finger, be reminded that your marriage is made of something even stronger and more beautiful." I exhaled deeply, talking to the image of wedding-day dad: "Well, what should I be reminded of when this symbol of beauty and strength breaks right down the middle?"

I exhaled again and then again, hoping to dissipate these brutal thoughts and the rising swell of tears. I held the two half-circle pieces in my palm, their new edges sharp. My heart shuddered. Was this somehow a sign that my wife and our marriage were now shattered forever? And then, it was as if I heard that same wedding-day dad say, "She may be broken, but you're going to help put her back together again."

Around that same time, about twenty-five hundred miles away, our families began making frantic preparations to travel to LA. My in-laws in Athens, Georgia, had called their close doctor friend, desperate for some information and advice to better understand the severity of Katherine's diagnosis and what they should do. This doctor instantly knew that bleeding in the brain near the brain stem was a matter of life-and-death. "Any matter with a daughter is serious," he told them calmly but earnestly. "You should go to her now."

My mother-in-law raced to catch the next cross-country flight heading west. My dad in Montgomery, Alabama, began similarly moving to catch a flight out of Atlanta, more than two hours away. A pair of his friends offered to get him there. On the high-speed ride, Dad called his doctor friend, a neurosurgeon, who more bluntly assessed the situation: "The laws of nature will have to be suspended in order for Katherine to survive."

As the hours passed, the crowd in vigil for Katherine grew and grew until nearly a hundred souls gathered in that hospital waiting room. There were tears and hushed whispers, but there were also bursts of laughter and aromas of pizza and quiet singing. That underwhelming space, with its chipped paint and stained rug and cracked armrests, began to metamorphose into something altogether different. In the gathering and in the praying and in the breaking of bread (or crust, as it were), the common elements were transubstantiated into a holy experience, as holy as any ancient cathedral or Communion because they were offered, not in the absence of suffering, but right in the midst of it.

The sun set, and the crowd flowed outside to the attached courtyard for some fresh air and prayer together. I lingered inside for a moment, gripping a battered crimson Gideon's Bible as if my life depended on it. Having grown up in a large church, I was accustomed to engaging a crowd for an extended period of time, but it was taking a toll on my natural introvert tendencies. Nonetheless, it was a wonderful distraction from the clock, which seemed to move so slowly that I actually thought it might have been broken. The surgery was scheduled to last eight hours, and the time could not pass quickly enough. If I stopped talking or moving too long, my mind instantly tortured me with a horrifying slideshow of the bloody scene unfolding in the operating room a few floors below. As our thoughts tend to do, mine refused to be tamed unless I distracted myself or until I finally remembered to pray those thoughts away.

I unconsciously flipped through the pages of that dog-eared Bible, wondering whose tears had fallen on its pages, whose hands had held it looking for comfort and answers. My eyes landed on the book of Romans, and I turned to the eighth chapter, Katherine's favorite. According to family lore, when Amie was young, she was required to memorize some verses from Romans 8. Not to be outdone by her little sister, Katherine, the perpetual firstborn, took it upon herself to memorize the whole chapter.

"I consider that our present sufferings are not worth comparing with the glory that will be revealed in us."

As I read the words, a strange conflict torqued my insides. I had never read this passage in a context like my present experience—one of real suffering, one that seemed devoid of anything good.

"And we know in all things, God works for the good of those who love him, who have been called according to his purpose."

The brokenness of that moment, of all the broken moments of creation, tremored down my spine, opening my eyes, as if for the first time, to the reality of this world. *How, God, could this be true? How could there be any good in this thing?*

Looking up from the pages, I glanced through the waiting-room window to the patio filled with my people, circled up, hands linked, praying. Earlier that day, word of Katherine's stroke spread like wildfire on social media and through emails and telephone chains. We would later learn that people all over the world were praying for Katherine, some unexplainably roused from sleep in the middle of the night, prompted to pray again while her surgery continued. Could there be a more comforting thought than knowing you are being prayed for when your own prayers have been stretched to their breaking point?

I joined the group outside, the California night pleasantly cool, the tall evergreens silhouetted against the bright moon and stars. We were all praying—pleading with God, comforted by the sureness of His grace, and wincing at the thought of Katherine's pain. As that time came to a close, I stood in front of the group and thanked them for their presence, assuring them that I felt anything but alone. I opened that well-used Bible and began reading the whole chapter of Romans 8. As the passage climaxed at the thirty-eighth verse, my voice faltered. My throat seized up so hard that I could barely even swallow. Hot tears filled my eyes and splashed down on the page below. I knew I could either obligatorily just read these words, or I could actually try to believe them, believe them so fervently as to stake everything on them—my life and Katherine's too. My voice returned, and I read these words with a new sense of peace.

"For I am convinced that neither death nor life, neither angels nor demons, neither the present nor the future, nor any powers, neither height nor depth, nor anything else in all creation, will be able to separate us from the love of God that is in Christ Jesus our Lord."

In that moment, I released Katherine from my feeble grip and into God's. I knew that, though Katherine may well lose her life, she would never lose the indomitable goodness and inexplicable love of God. And neither would I.

Several shifts of anesthesiologists and assistants came and went during what turned out to be sixteen hours of surgery. As the sun arose over the courtyard, the crowd had whittled to just a handful when the weary neurosurgeon approached.

"Katherine lived," he said quietly. "It is nothing short of a miracle."

A collective smile rose from our mouths while tears of gratitude welled up in our squinty eyes. This was the answer we had spent the whole night waiting for.

"But we don't know what the deficits will be," he added, not wanting to squelch our relief but also not wanting to miscommunicate the current state of affairs. He explained that Kathcrinc had had a hemorrhagic stroke, a bleed in her brain, because of the rupture of an Arterial Venous Malformation (AVM), a congenital condition that causes an abnormal collection of blood vessels. As a person ages, these thin-walled vessels can expand and break, causing a hemorrhage into the brain. Katherine's brain stem was completely engulfed in blood, and the massive pressure from the bleeding was literally squeezing her brain down into her spine. Although the surgery had gone very well, Dr. Gonzalez knew that multiple intracranial ncrvcs were sacrificed in order to save Katherine's life, likely resulting in paralysis of the face and swallowing reflex and possible impairment of her hearing, eyesight, and speech. More horrifying than that, there was a possibility that Katherine might be completely paralyzed and left in a vegetative state. In the span of a day, we went from living an idyllic, carefree life in Malibu to having life as we'd known it hanging by the thinnest thread.

The air went out of the room as my mother-in-law shrieked and fell back into her chair, wailing. But Katherine was alive. I hugged Dr. Gonzalez, squeezing this virtual stranger as if he was my long-lost relative. "Thank you. Thank you," I murmured. No other words came, because no other words would suffice.

At that moment, as the sun arose, unveiling a new day and a new life for all in that room, something began to rise in my heart too. During the seemingly endless night, I had struggled with the unbelievable prospect that I may well be a twenty-six-year-old widower and single dad by morning, that April 22 might be a new world—one without Katherine. Awash in relief that Katherine had lived, I felt sure that despite the terrifying possibilities of her future and the unknowns of her recovery, one thing was sure: God had spared her life for a reason.

As the crowds flowed into the halls of the hospital that morning, it seemed like just another normal day for everyone but us. Groggily, I staggered around the waiting room, which was now refilled with new friends arriving to show their support. I was reunited with James, who had been watched through the night by our dear friends, Ryan and Sarah. They all slept on the floor of another friend's office at UCLA. They could hardly sleep at the thought that this baby would likely wake up to a new world, one without a mother. I squeezed him hard and stared into his eyes, taking inventory of this precious little life, tracing his fingers and arms, ears and mouth—all of which reminded me of Katherine more than anything else on earth. I fed him a bottle for the first time ever, not totally sure of how to do it. Katherine had exclusively breastfed him until the day before, and neither James nor I seemed very fond of this new, necessary arrangement. I held him tightly, not wanting to put him on the ground, back into this place of unexpected dangers and dying parents. Yet he wriggled from my grasp with an object in his sights, and I put him down with a sigh. I suppose to love someone well is to assure them you will never leave them and then to let them go.

In a great reversal moment, across the room, I saw my dad burst through the waiting room doors. It was as though I reverted back to a childlike state as I ran to him. The necessary defenses that had built up during the night I had endured all fell off. In his arms, I instantly began to cry like a scared child. We went back to the prayer chapel and wept together for a long time. There are few more viscerally transformational experiences than the secure embrace of a loving parent, especially when the child truly recognizes their need.

My dad comes from a long line of Texans, perhaps men who were not the first to weep but men who got things done and in whose hands you would entrust your life. And as a pastor, perhaps his most unique skill was walking the halls of hospitals and standing by gravesides and tenderly loving the sick and dying and hurting. I was totally spent in the deepest ways, emotionally and physically, but it was okay because he was there. And I would need him—his strength and his reassurances—for one of the more pivotal moments I would experience: seeing Katherine again.

Around midday, my mother-in-law, Dad, and I were invited to Katherine's ICU room. We took the elevator up to this different part of the hospital. There were no words to fill the tiny space churning with anticipation and terror. We watched the light methodically click up each floor until we arrived on 7. The lucky number. The number of completion. It felt anything but. We were buzzed into the ICU, a place awash with the same tumultuous mix of emotions from the elevator but now coupled with real-life images from our nightmares, set to a score of beeps and bellows from life-support machines, hushed whispers, and the deep sighs of loss. Katherine had been given one of the only actual rooms in the unit, rather than a shared space partitioned off by curtains. A full wall of windows connected her room to the nurses' station. It was as if she lay in a glass jewelry box or a museum, a rare specimen to be studied and treasured.

I breathed in deeply as we entered, and the strangely sweet smell of antiseptics mixed with bandages and blood is a smell I recall to this day. The scene before me was too unreal to process, and it was worse than the images my mind had conjured up that plagued me through the night. Katherine's body was swollen unrecognizably. Her face and head were unnaturally round like the moon and covered with white bandages, save for a matted mound of rust-colored hair and a shockingly exposed patch of now-shaved scalp right above her forehead, like the first pass of a lawn mower on an overgrown yard. From that bald strip, a tube protruded into her brain that helped to drain the unwanted blood presently mingled with her cerebrospinal fluid. That tube entwined with nearly a dozen other wires and tubes connecting this body to the machines that were literally giving it life. Her eyes were shut, and her lips were pursed and cracked around the respirator tube, which was affixed to her face with strips of tape, like a child's attempt to repair a favorite broken doll. Her expression was neither pained nor peaceful. It was empty. She was still, save for the sickeningly rhythmic rising and falling of her chest by the life-support machine.

Nausea and bewilderment welled up as if I was in the severest descent on a roller coaster, and I fell to the floor, reaching up to the bed with one hand, not knowing where to touch or whom I was even touching. The juxtaposition of the nearly lifeless Katherine I was seeing and the vital, energetic woman I had known was too much to take in. Katherine had always been my grounding, my call home, my reminder of who I was. Yet the Katherine I had known and loved, the Katherine I had laughed and cried with, married, and had a child with, was nowhere to be found.

I fumbled around the sheets for her hand and placed mine on top of hers. There was no reassuring squeeze. It was cold and

nearly lifeless. Yet along the sides of her thumb, I felt the familiar roughness from years of nervous nibbling when she was
stressed, just like her dad. We had tried to break the habit, but
to no avail. This place that was once perhaps her "most broken"
spot was now by far her least broken one. I traced the polish-
chipped nail and rubbed her thumb like a rabbit's foot, like an
Ebenezer stone. And I remembered it was her, my Katherine.

By day's end, more family and friends had arrived, some dropping
everything to fly across the country and give us the costly gift
of their physical presence. One such friend came from Alabama
to California, suspending his high-powered attorney world to
accomplish a simple mission—to "encourage the encouragers."
The waiting-room crowd waxed like an ocean tide as people got
out of work and came straight to the hospital, and church small
groups shifted their meeting place from their living rooms to
the hospital waiting room. My in-laws were reunited, mourning
this unimaginable turn of events for their eldest daughter, and
when evening came, they left, exhausted.

I could barely muster any more strength to engage the
crowd, let alone absorb the reality of Katherine's current state. I
was haunted by the stark contrast in encountering the most life-
filled person I had ever known now absolutely devoid of life. It
seemed a shameful defeat, but I asked my dad and his friend to
be my proxy and go back up to the ICU to tell Katherine good
night for me, because I could not.

As night fell, it seemed my hope was slowly being overcome
by the same darkness engulfing the world outside the waiting-
room windows. In comparison to the unsinkable feeling sparked
in my soul as the sun had risen that morning, I was succumbing
to the doubts and fears that swirled around me like a riptide,
threatening to drag me down to the bottom of an ocean of grief.

From the corner of my eye, I saw my dad running. My stomach dropped, and I turned my head in slow motion, scared of what I might see. He was smiling, almost giddily, motioning for me to come with him. "Katherine is responding to the nurse's commands!" I followed him back up the elevator in childlike wonder and confusion, hardly knowing what he meant. We burst back into the ICU, disregarding the clear preparations being made for sleep. We crowded close around the bed, waiting with bated breath, as if the nurse was going to perform the greatest magic trick we had ever seen. She swiftly removed the bottom part of the sheet covering Katherine's feet while I prayed silently, *Please, God, I can't bear the prospect of hope if I'm just going to be let down.*

"Katherine, honey, if you can hear me, wiggle your toes," the nurse commanded softly. I slowly turned my gaze to the foot of the bed and beheld the most glorious sight I had ever seen . . . Katherine's toes wiggling and rippling like a flag in the wind! It was as jaw-dropping as any magic trick ever performed, because it was real.

"Katherine, your family is here. Honey, Jay is here. He's been so worried about you. Can you show him how you can lift your fingers too?" Like the slight, first motions of a marionette puppet, her left hand rose, fingers making a peace sign, as if lifted by invisible string. Seeing that subtle sign of hope made me feel like a drain was pulled from my body as the black water of fear and despair that had been filling my insides began to rapidly drain away. Whimpering laughs and tears of amazement and gratitude rose from us all.

Katherine was supposed to be in a medically induced coma for days, and yet, a little more than twelve hours after her surgery, she was already straining to come back to us—a sign of her grit and an assurance of God's grace. This little movement, sparked from an external command that she heard and processed, meant she was not paralyzed or brain-dead. The mundane simplicity of the action belied its stunningly miraculous nature: It meant life, and even the smallest sign is the beginning of hope.

Understandably exhausted after the operation, Dr. Gonzales had already gone home to bed, and under such circumstances, the ICU nursing staff would not normally dare to disturb him. But when they awakened him with this stunning news, he was incredulous—so much so that he rushed back to the hospital to see for himself what he (and everyone else) thought was a medical impossibility. Dr. Gonzalez got tears in his eyes when he did a cursory neurological exam and Katherine squeezed his hand. He said that as incredibly well as the surgery went, he couldn't take credit for such miraculous outcomes. He'd had "a helper," he said, pointing up.

A constant stream of friends continued to surround us. The OR waiting room was quickly becoming a gathering place, like the neighborhood hangout where your name and usual order are already known. One friend noted that no matter when she came to that waiting room, before or after work, during the day or late at night, someone was always there with a shared hope with whom she could commune. It was like the best version of church for her. This simple room had taken on an unearthly, holy quality to those of us who gathered for the common purpose of walking together through this suffering.

Mia, our beloved, graphic designer friend, created a large-scale sign designating the area that our group had inadvertently claimed as "Katherine's Corner." Though Katherine was no longer in the operating room, this OR waiting area was the only one that could contain our large crowds that came to sit in extended vigil. We sat mingled among families of patients waiting, as we had waited, for their loved ones in surgery. There is an instant closeness, a camaraderie that springs from the shared experience of pain; yet in acute circumstances, we are often, quite naturally, self-focused. The amazing thing for us was that because we were not actually waiting for the end of a surgery, we were free to come alongside those who were.

I remember sitting next to a woman whose body jerked upright at the sight of her husband's doctor approaching. I watched with vicarious breathlessness, anticipating the news he would deliver. From afar, his somber face already seemed to communicate the result. I saw the woman's shoulders began to heave, and I suddenly wished I could have been anywhere but there. Yet such is the waiting room. There is nowhere to quickly hide from your own pain or the pain of others; it must be experienced and shared together. Realizing his unfortunate choice of facial expression, the doctor blurted out, "Your husband's just fine. He did great in the surgery!" The woman's tears came still, but now, they were tears of joy. And mine came too. We all walk through this life on the edge of a blade, and yet we rarely allow ourselves to feel the weight of our potential losses or the grace of our potential gains. I offered my tear-filled congratulations to her, and we shared a familial hug.

The food began to pour in, as happens during any crisis. A large cooler was dragged to our designated corner of the waiting room, as if in preparation for some tailgating festivities preceding a NASCAR race, except the beer and chicken wings were replaced with green juice and gluten-free energy bars—this is California, after all. We were later asked to remove said cooler for health code reasons, to which we offered the kindly volunteer a cold beverage, thus buying a few more days of her looking the other way. Pizzas were delivered to the waiting room like a frat house. One day, a bag of foot-long sub sandwiches was dropped off simultaneous with a ten-pack of large matzo ball soups (from Katherine's acting teacher). Feeling anything but hungry, I offered these to our group, and having few takers,

I charged everyone with handing out the food to our fellow waiting-room residents.

It's amazing how free food can drop human defenses like few things in this world. Our offerings in hand, we were invited to sit with people—scared people—and give them something that might help sustain their bodies as well as something that might help sustain their souls . . . our story of hope. Though we were only a few steps ahead of them in our hospital experience, there was already an ownership and a call to action that we all felt. We had seen something miraculous in the circumstances surrounding Katherine's stroke and survival, and we felt compelled to share what had been given to us with others in need.

I sat down by a large group to offer them some food, which they accepted, and in return, they told me their story. This group was tight-knit, yet in the throes of real pain as they waited. The family's beloved matriarch had fallen ill while hosting Shabbat dinner for her family. She had retired early and had surprisingly declined to an almost unresponsive state by the next day. Like us, within the course of a few hours, they had found their world turned completely upside down. The mom was in her early sixties. We quickly determined that she now lay in the seventh-floor ICU room adjacent to Katherine's. Our bond instantly deepened, and I promised to pray for them and be of any help I could. Later in the day as I returned to the ICU, I glimpsed their mother through a sliver of curtain, and my heart longed for her restoration as if she was my own mother.

Our church community created a schedule by which at least one person would be in the OR waiting room twenty-four hours a day, literally spending the entire night on the floor, watching for any change, offering any aid. Most of them never even got to see Katherine in the ICU, but nonetheless they came, offering their prayers and presence to us and to others they encountered there. It was an inestimable gift to know that just a few floors below Katherine was someone watching and waiting for her around the clock. This stunning offering continued for three weeks straight until we finally convinced them that this specific vigil could come to an end.

As we progressed through all the pain together and found God in the midst, we were surprised to find that our hearts did not have to shrink in self-defense. Rather, as our hearts were filled to overflowing with the comfort we so desperately needed, our bourgeoning hope could spill out onto those in need. We who were the receivers became the givers, and in so giving, we were continually refilled and encouraged by the realization that none of our suffering would be wasted.

The sight of blood has always made my wrists tingle. Yet I was presented with the reality that this hospital would be my new home, and blood would be a rather constant companion. I had, of course, heard of someone having a stroke—maybe someone's grandmother—but I knew very little about the ins and outs of this diagnosis. As helpless and underqualified as I felt, Katherine's rally in responding to commands the night after her surgery empowered me. I had to force aside my shortcomings and stand by her, even in the midst of the hospital smells and all the blood. I wanted, more than anything, for Katherine to know she was not fighting this greatest fight of her life alone.

On April 23, only two days after her stroke, Katherine opened her eyes for the first time. Clearly, a medically induced coma didn't mean what it used to, at least not to Katherine. She was not going to take this event lying down. I suppose I expected a scene out of a movie, where the sick patient weakly but serenely opens her eyes to the loved ones gathered around the bedside. What I did see was out of a different kind of movie. Katherine's bright blue eyes were intact, but they spun shockingly in their sockets like nothing I have ever seen, dramatically rolling like marbles in a glass until they settled. The right eye, however, settled unnaturally, turned in and down, as if afraid of what it might see, while the left eye stayed in its normal, assigned position, seeming to take in everything in the room.

I spent that first night Katherine was awake in the room with her. Her eyes, though not under her control, looked at me with a clear sense of fear and longing. I didn't know what to tell her besides, "You are safe here," though I wondered if I believed it. All around us were sick and dying people, all suffering from similar brain-related maladies. As Katherine's late doctor-grandfather was known to say, "A hospital is no place for sick people." While sleep was encouraged, it was simultaneously prevented by a constant routine of checking vitals and emptying urine bags. I tried to stay awake as long as possible, but found myself exhaustedly slumping down in a chair, laying my head on the bed next to Katherine's leg, holding her hand.

I awoke to the still-dark room and hushed but urgent voices tending to the tube protruding from Katherine's head. The ventriculostomy tube connecting the inside of her brain to a meter by her bedside was both the most horrific sight and yet one of the most necessary pieces on her new machinized body. Its purpose was to measure intracranial pressure and aid her currently impaired cerebrospinal fluid circulation. If this simple system showed an increase in pressure, Katherine's responsiveness would delay noticeably, or worse, she would become completely nonresponsive.

I felt like I was in the way as the team gathered around her to assess the problem. I apologetically stood up and walked out of her room through waves of nausea from lack of sleep and witnessing them "tapping the brain shunt" to unclog it. "O God, I can't do this," I whispered. I slumped against the wall and slid down to the floor in the empty hallway. And yet a realization came quickly: *Katherine can't do this either—not by herself.*

The next night, I opted to sleep in an actual bed at a hotel across the street, but I was awakened at about 3:00 a.m. by the buzz of my cell phone. My heart immediately began pounding out of my chest as I stuttered out a terrified "Hello?"

"Your wife seems to want you," said the ICU nurse.

I threw on some clothes and raced across the street in the cool air of predawn. As I arrived by her bed, her left eye signaled relief at my presence. "She hasn't been able to sleep at all," the nurse informed me. I tried to imagine the claustrophobia she must be feeling, and it made me tear up. "It's okay, Katherine. You can go to sleep now. I'll be right here." With that, she closed her eyes, opening them a few more times just to see if I was still there.

I opened a Bible from her bedside table and read through Romans again. Then I flipped to Job, a book I had honestly hardly ever read before because it seemed like kind of a downer.

The story opens with these words: "In the land of Uz there lived a man whose name was Job. This man was blameless and upright; he feared God and shunned evil."

I couldn't help but superimpose Katherine's name there . . .

"In the City of Angeles there lived a woman whose name was Katherine. This woman was blameless and upright; she feared God and shunned evil."

I read through the entire book in the same way. This most ancient of biblical texts felt so strikingly modern, so relevant to Katherine's story, that I was stunned. I considered the reality that sometimes suffering comes because of the decisions we make; sometimes it comes as a way for God to gauge His place in our hearts; and sometimes it comes simply as a by-product of living in a world that is in a state of falling apart. Yet no matter the origin of the suffering, God's presence remains the same. He finds us in our hurts, if we want to be found. His power to filter the worst that life has to offer, with goodness remaining, is our great hope.

But then, four chapters later, after Job's horrendous suffering has been recounted, I read these words, and the hairs on my arm stood on end: "For he wounds, but he also binds up; he injures, but his hands also heal."

This picture of God was one I had never considered before. The words caught me off guard, stinging deeply as their reality sunk into my soul. If God is all-powerful and all-knowing, and thus could have stopped this but did not, then He is in some way culpable. "God, why would You allow all this suffering to come into Katherine's life? God, how could You wound her so deeply? Why? WHY?"

I began to cry in a way I never had before, muffling my sobs so as not to wake up the finally sleeping patient. It was an anguished, prayerful weeping, not just for Katherine, but for all the "Katherines." I felt like a whimpering, bewildered child, not crying for lost toys, but crying at the first realization that life wasn't fair, that nothing was safe. Having grown up in a large church, I had encountered much loss and pain in the lives of church members. My dad would have to leave the dinner table to make an emergency hospital visit or counsel someone in crisis. He presided over hundreds of funerals, some for children. We were not shielded from this, for which I am grateful, and yet it created a sense of resignation, a drought of tears, a hardening of the heart. That night in Katherine's room, a deluge of tears bathed my heart, dissolving its shell of stone, revealing a heart of flesh. And it hurt deeply to feel everything, as if for the first time. Yet as I wiped away my tears and snot and spit, I seemed to find more of myself underneath, and I seemed to find more of God there too.

Suddenly, my heartbreak at the revelation of God's apparent complicity in Katherine's tragedy shifted. As I scanned her broken body, full of new cracks and pins and tubes, I realized that these were all made by her doctors and nurses as they sought to save her life. They had horrifically wounded her in brain surgery and ICU so that she might be healed. I sat with this thought, the confounding complexity of which overcame me so much that I closed my eyes and prayed, "O God, I can't begin to understand what You're doing, but maybe Your paradoxes aren't as paradoxical as they seem. If You have been part of her wounding, then You must be part of her healing."

I awoke soon thereafter, the room still dark, though slightly illuminated by the artificial starlight of machines scattered around her bed. I could make out the silhouette of her body against the lightening horizon outside the window, the familiarity of her profile and frame evident despite the wild hair and addition of tubes and wires that looked like a child's handmade headdress of sticks and feathers. Suddenly, I noticed small pinpoints of golden light appear, dotting Katherine's body at the places where IVs and respirators and shunts now pierced her skin. I gazed in wonder as the warm lights began to flicker and grow, soon overwhelming her darkened figure with kinetic golden streams flowing from her broken places, commingling and filling the room and hospital and then overflowing like a radiant, living wave onto the city outside. It was a surreal vision, a waking dream, a stark reminder that perhaps in the breaking of precious things, something even more precious than we can imagine might be unleashed. Perhaps in the breaking, we can find the healing we long for.

Katherine was a model patient in the ICU. I was surprised to encounter so many families and patients who were in such pain and acted out of that hurt toward the medical professionals caring for them. I was guilty of it too, but I was inspired to follow Katherine's lead as she wordlessly connected with and comforted those who were helping her. Her veins were so weak and overstrained that it took four different nurses to finally get an IV in her. They tried her arm, wrist, the back of her hand, and finally the top of her foot. I was nearly at my wit's end, about

to scream that these so-called professionals were worthless—
they couldn't even start an IV! Yet Katherine, in an unearthly
manner, extended her already bruised left arm to the flustered
nurse, who finally hit the mark. Katherine touched her with
such warmth and kindness that the nurse teared up. They all
knew that this young woman was living an absolute hell, but,
inexplicably, she was a picture of grace.

My sister Sarah had come from Ethiopia, where she was living as a missionary. She would soon resign from her position to
be part of James's full-time care team, which also included both
of our mothers and a village of friends. Katherine and I have
five sisters between us, three of whom were still in high school
at that time. Sarah and I are the closest in age, and it became a
unique time for us to reconnect through this great tragedy.

Katherine's room was filled with a constant hum of praise
music from a small bedside speaker—the same playlist Katherine
had on repeat during her labor and delivery with James. One
afternoon, a shrieking blood oxygen level alarm went off dozens
of times in the course of a few hours. A maddening cacophony of
sounds resulted from the alarm and music, so I finally turned off
the speaker in my annoyance.

In the moment of sudden peace, I decided that Sarah and I
would sing to Katherine ourselves instead, something we had
not done since childhood. Katherine had been given a unique
gift from a family friend, a strangely angled wooden cross, hand
carved to fit right in the holder's palm. This "holding cross"
stayed in Katherine's grip for weeks, a comforting sign that she
was holding on to Jesus with everything she had. As we sang,
she wordlessly voiced her delight, praising God in the most
poignant way, raising her left hand and the cross heavenward
as high as she could. It was hard to finish all the verses of her
favorite hymn, "Turn Your Eyes upon Jesus," in light of her
moving and heartfelt act of worship. The song would become
our anthem of sorts.

As we left the ICU each night, Sarah and I would take a side stairwell that opened to the exterior of the building, deeply breathing in the fresh night air. In a cathartic, meditative way, we would sing the hymn together, harmonizing effortlessly as the voices of siblings can do. In light of the horrors of the ICU we encountered daily, we needed to tell ourselves the same faith-filled story night after night. *"Turn your eyes upon Jesus, look full in His wonderful face, and the things of earth will grow strangely dim in the light of His glory and grace."* At the end of one particularly long night, our feet touched the ground floor just as we sang the final words, which echoed up the stairwell like the smoke of a burnt offering. Above us, we heard the sound of a single person's applause.

From the day of her stroke, there were amazing words of encouragement, even prophetic visions and vibrant dreams had by people from all over the world. Dozens of people recounted that as they prayed for Katherine, they felt strongly drawn to the story of Jairus's daughter, raised from the dead by Jesus as recorded in Mark 5. In verse 41, Jesus commands her, *"Talitha koum"*—which means, "Little girl, get up!" And she does. In so many ways, this verse had been prophetic in Katherine's life. She had been all but dead, and yet God miraculously gave her life again. Nonetheless, these striking promises were a double-edged sword. Many people believed with all their hearts that Katherine would be healed so miraculously that she would be getting up out of her hospital bed in no time, just like the little girl did. As the weeks passed with only microscopic improvements, the recounting of those visions began to dry up, and these beautiful visuals, encouraging me to press on and to press into a God who raises the dead, suddenly felt like a lie.

A friend of mine from law school asked if she could visit Katherine in the ICU. They did not know each other well, but this friend tentatively recounted that she had been involved in two instances where she laid her hands on sick people and they were healed. I was honestly a bit skeptical but figured we had nothing to lose. Did I not have enough faith that God could do this? Did I not believe that Katherine could be miraculously healed in her physical body?

My friend nervously entered the room and placed her hands gently on Katherine's right arm and leg. I stood on Katherine's other side, following my friend's lead as she prayed. Perhaps I was expecting something with laser lights to happen, or at the very least something in the same vein as a charismatic tent revival. But when I opened my eyes, I looked down on the same broken body hooked up to the same machines. I didn't know how much Katherine was internalizing all this or how much her hopes for a miraculous healing had been lifted and then dashed. I didn't know what to say, but I thanked my friend for her time, despite the fact that her healing average had been taken down a notch. I did want Katherine to be well, to be healed, to get out of the hospital and go back to being a mom and being my wife. I wanted that as desperately as I have ever wanted anything. But I felt in my soul that the way and the time in which Katherine would be healed was not up to me.

One night, I shared these thoughts with my mom. In the expressing of my desire for Katherine's healing, it was clear that part of my desire for it came from my own deep need. I had lost the old Katherine, and I wanted a new one, even if she was different. I was starting to have trouble even remembering the sound of her voice when she said my name, or how she smelled after a shower, or the feel of the small of her back when we danced. There was an almost frantic grasping for a memory of the woman I loved. But they all were fading fast as I was constantly inundated with the very different sights and smells and sounds and touches associated with this new Katherine.

The questions remained. *What does it mean to be healed? Was this a test of faith, and if so, was I failing? Was everyone who was praying for Katherine failing?* These thoughts reverberated in my head like a broken record. *Could all these people who had seen visions of a restored Katherine be wrong? Are they lying to me, or is God lying to them?* A comforting and terrifying thought remained: *Maybe healing just looks different than we think it does.* Maybe Katherine will be healed in a way we could recognize and celebrate. But maybe she had already been healed as much as she would be—and if so, was that enough healing for me?

⚓

Katherine could not speak because she had a tracheostomy in her throat, connecting her to the respirator. But her left eye and, amazingly, her left hand began to increasingly communicate volumes. The vigor with which she would normally speak seemed to have migrated to her once-weakened left hand, which now moved at an almost comically fast speed compared to the near lifelessness of the rest of her body. She would gesture ecstatically in response to questions and even created her own makeshift version of sign language, with the universal sign for James being her hand cupping and squeezing invisible, chunky baby thighs.

I became a quick student of the ICU, not only learning the medical terms and procedures but also getting to know the people who worked there. They became friends, maybe out of pity, or maybe because I brought them cupcakes to show my thanks and would genuinely ask them how they were doing. These small kindnesses afforded all of Katherine's supporters some special privileges. The normal visiting hours didn't seem to apply to us, and we were even able to sneak James up to see his mommy a few times a week.

May 11, only three weeks after the stroke, was Mother's Day, and it was Katherine's first as a mom herself. Anna had dressed James in a onesie with a bold red "MOM" on the front, and I wrangled him unwillingly up the elevator to give his mom the only gift she wanted that day—a moment with her baby. The scene was one almost too painful to bear. I held back tears at the sight of James, oblivious to the fact that the figure in the bed on which he sat was his mother. The ventriculostomy tube was still prominently sprouting from her head, and plastic wrap now covered half her face to protect her right eye, which was exposed due to her facial paralysis. James did not seem to recognize her, yet there was no fear either, for which I was grateful. She groped around for his leg and found his thigh. A slight smile crept up the left side of her face as James smiled too.

One of Katherine's nurses told us that the ICU team referred to Katherine as "our miracle girl." The nurse had just returned from a two-week vacation and said, "Katherine's progress is miraculous. After seeing the severity of her trauma, her improvement is so encouraging that it makes me glad to come to work." She went on to say that UCLA's neurological unit sees many patients who are severely injured, and generally the medical team accurately predicts a very bleak outcome. "However, Katherine has beaten the odds," the nurse said, "and her comeback has been so good for us. Her progress has lifted the spirits of the whole team!"

The CEO of the hospital had deemed Katherine's case a "new paradigm for patient support," as not only was the physical presence of her supporters incredibly large, but the digital interest in her story was also so great that a link to the hospital's website from Katherine's online prayer update page crashed UCLA's computer servers.

Yet surprisingly, some members of the ICU didn't really care who we were or what kind of miracle they were encountering. They knew the rules, and they were not bending them. Fair enough. One such ICU aide was quick to snap at any of my visits outside normal hours and any requests outside normal regulations. At first, I felt almost irrationally angry at this woman who didn't know my situation and didn't seem to care to know it. It seemed she might use her small amount of power to derail my important mission with Katherine.

One night, as I was complaining to myself about the aide's irrational rudeness, our nurse asked me if I wanted them to fully shave Katherine's hair, as it seemed irreparably matted with blood from her surgery, like a horrific set of dreadlocks from hell. Without hesitation, I instructed the nurse to shave Katherine's head so she could start afresh. My mother-in-law, also without hesitation, piped in with something to the effect of "over my dead body will you shave my baby's head." The Arnold girls were known for their long, blonde manes, and as Katherine now looked so different from her previous self, her mom concluded that keeping the long hair was perhaps the last vestige of a different life, a life where things like hair upkeep actually made the list of important tasks. I rolled my eyes and shot back, "Well, I'm not going to be the one trying to brush out those tangles, Kim. Good luck with that."

I arrived the next morning still ruffled and on the defensive after the events of the previous evening. When I entered Katherine's room, I let out a gasp of disbelief. During the night, Katherine had received an ambush makeover of sorts. Her hair was no longer thrown into a disheveled, bloody bun, but rather it was washed and combed through, tightly gathered at the top of her head in a slick braid. This very fair-skinned blonde girl now had the appearance of an exotic Latina genie. I liked it.

My ICU aide nemesis walked around the corner with the nurse and, much to my surprise, explained that they had spent nearly four hours untangling Katherine's hair piece by piece, brushing out the knots with the help of a little morphine and then lovingly washing it in their makeshift ICU salon (aka a clean bedpan). They finished the look with the aide's signature braid, the same one she did on her little girls' hair every day. She even added a sparkly scrunchie, like a neon cherry on top.

I approached the woman, my anger evaporating completely. Though not Katherine's typical coiffure, there was an unexpected sense of empowerment in her new hairdo and a sense of dignity that I had not seen since her arrival in the ICU.

I was overcome with a deep sense of humility as I hugged the aide and thanked her for loving Katherine so well and for communicating to Katherine, in a way I had not, that she was worth the untangling of every knot.

Those first weeks in the ICU were wrought with drama, each day ending with a new cliff-hanger begging the question, "Will she make it through this too?" That tense twisting and turning quality to the unfolding events made our story instantly engaging to a surprising legion of dedicated strangers and friends alike. At that time, many digital forms of story sharing were just peaking in their availability to the masses. We later found out that in the days following the stroke, multiple blogs and Facebook groups popped up, unbeknownst to us, calling this digital audience to pray on Katherine's behalf, and on the main medical/prayer website created by a friend of ours, hits were tracked from 120 countries, numbering in the tens of thousands of unique visitors. The response was overwhelming, so we continued to share all the needs for prayer, all the doubts, and all the hopes to these invisible cheerleaders.

We candidly shared the array of horrific but necessary medical procedures performed on Katherine in the ICU. New prayers were needed for each of these daily. She underwent dangerous angiograms to check on the status of her postsurgical brain and to treat potentially deadly vasospasms, which are akin to brain-wide ministrokes. She also had more permanent IV ports installed, along with a tracheostomy and gastrostomy tube, tragically signifying the reality of much longer-term inabilities to breathe or eat on her own. The right side of her face was paralyzed, including her eyelid, leaving her right eye exposed, resulting in a corneal tear. Lack of body movement, nonexistent swallowing, and artificial respiration were the perfect trifecta for pneumonia, which she contracted multiple times. As she had been breastfeeding up to the day of her stroke, she was engorged and suffered a terrible infection and fever from mastitis. They had to bind her chest like a Shakespearean female actor in order to stop the production of breast milk. This too was a somber sign that she would not be returning to her normal motherly duties anytime soon. Perhaps the most horrifying procedure was the Cool Guard, a system that lowered her overall body temperature by effectively running sterile iced saline through her veins. This helped combat the high fevers brought on from multiple infections and also created a better environment for her brain to heal. Katherine *hates* to be cold, so the sight of her shivering and convulsing violently in response to this inescapable cold was torturous to watch.

We chose this level of vulnerability in our communication with others, in spite of hesitation from some family and friends on the effect of this type of exposure, because we knew we needed all the prayers and support we could get. We hoped that in the sharing, we would somehow open our tragedy to the light and not feel so alone in our pain. This was for our own benefit, but also for the benefit of those encountering it. In the letters, emails, and comments we received, it soon became apparent that the sharing of our story of hope was opening up the possibility that hope might come into the painful stories of our readers as well.

My dad and mother-in-law both shared their uniquely different interpretations of Katherine's medical events to their respective readers, often finding themselves at opposite ends of the spectrum in terms of how they were processing the same story. It was challenging to find a middle ground that was able to both mourn the loss of so much and at the same time to yearn toward a hopeful outcome. This juxtaposition reminded me that as much as this story intersected the lives of our families, it was, at the end of the day, Katherine's story and mine and James's, and it was one that we needed to figure out how to tell ourselves.

Despite the roller coaster of emotions and the endlessly compounding obstacles against her, I knew deeply, undoubtedly that Katherine would get out of that hospital and that she would live her life again. The best man in our wedding was getting married that August, and I was supposed to be in the wedding. I even went with my mom and sisters to buy the specified groomsman suit at the mall near the hospital. I fully envisioned Katherine and me both attending—Katherine holding on to my arm, maybe looking a little weak but just like her old self, even wearing high heels as we walked down the aisle, smiling at each other triumphantly.

Whether it was shock or some other subconscious, self-preservation mechanism, I was certainly naive to the reality of what it looks like to survive and recover from the type of injury from which she had suffered. Of course, I knew she had undergone sixteen hours of surgery and the AVM had been removed and some vital nerves and functions were sacrificed in order to save her life. Nevertheless, I felt so confused when I heard a nurse summarizing Katherine's case to the next nurse at shift change: "Subarachnoid hemorrhage, necessitating a craniectomy and laminectomy, with resectioning of AVM and removal of 60 percent of the cerebellum . . ."

I interjected quizzically, "Removal? What do you mean removal?" In our shock, no one had asked for a blow-by-blow explanation of what exactly happened to Katherine in surgery. I don't think we could have fully processed it if it had been explained early on.

Dr. Gonzales later told us that Katherine's AVM was the largest he had ever seen, in the worst possible location, and with the worst possible amount of bleeding. The AVM was in her right cerebellum, which sits at the base of the brain and closest to the spinal cord. Dr. Gonzales had to perform a craniectomy (removing the back right portion of Katherine's skull) as well as a laminectomy (removing several of her top vertebral bones) to give her swelling brain a little more room to expand. During the first half of the surgery, he worked painstakingly on her brain to separate healthy blood vessels from those he had discovered were damaged beyond repair. He removed the AVM—and with it, over half of Katherine's cerebellum. The surgery involved so much bleeding that her full blood volume was replaced five times. We were told she had been given 10 percent of all the blood used at the UCLA Medical Center that day!

Somehow the idea that something had been removed from Katherine's body, something vital, something that had been a part of her for twenty-six years, hit me hard. Katherine was somehow irreparably different. My fantastical visions of her resurrected, blemishless body began to seem embarrassingly childish, impossible even. It was the beginning of a growing realization that Katherine would never be the same again. While she was still physically alive, it was clear that the old Katherine had, in fact, died and would never be coming back.

Nearly a month into her ICU stay, she was deemed stable enough to engage her first session of physical therapy. This seemed crazy, as she was still connected to a respirator, not to mention multiple IVs, tubes, and cords. A motionless body quickly falls victim to one of nature's most basic laws: entropy. This deterioration was evident in the twenty pounds she had lost, most of it muscle. Her legs and arms were becoming skeletal. The next phase of her healing would require her to muster strength her body did not have in order to stop its further deterioration. It seemed an almost impossible Catch-22.

Physical therapy (PT) in the ICU is quite different than in less acute contexts. That first session required no less than three people, including myself, to make sure Katherine's head and neck were supported and the necessary tubes were gathered and would not be pulled out as we lifted her like a life-sized ventriloquist doll to the edge of her hospital bed. The strain of this simple motion was evident as her eyes rolled in their sockets and her mouth hung, saliva dripping, almost corpse-like, the sight of which was so pitiful that I rushed to close her mouth. Her left eye suddenly looked at me in a moment of almost childlike shame. Bashfully, she struggled to not let her mouth unhinge again. My hopes for this to be her first time standing or walking were shattered, as merely sitting up on the edge of her bed, fully supported by others, was nearly enough to do her in for the rest of the day.

Nevertheless, Katherine continued to improve. Her blood pressure returned to normal, reducing the danger of deadly vasospasms. Her intracranial pressure was low, which meant her cerebrospinal fluid was circulating well. Her time on the respirator was being gradually reduced, which prompted her to do more breathing on her own. She had a "moderated cough," which indicated that the cough/gag/swallow reflex was improving—a vital part of the equation in getting her off the breathing machine. The Cool Guard was removed after nine consecutive days of misery.

Her miraculous improvement continued to encourage those who were following our story. One day, one of Katherine's ICU nurses brought her a gift—a beautiful blanket quilted by the young nurse's mother. More beautiful than the quilt was the accompanying note from this kind mom. "Katherine, as I read the web pages about your terrible journey, God has profoundly changed something in my heart. My faith has returned. While you have been lying in a bed of suffering, you have helped me arise."

⚓

While Katherine was in ICU, I was set to graduate from Pepperdine's law school. I honestly could not have cared less about going to the ceremony, but both of our families were in town and encouraged me to go, particularly since it had only been officially confirmed a few days before that I could even graduate at all.

Katherine's stroke occurred before I had taken my first final of the last semester. There had been weeks of dispute as to how this should be handled, and it was suggested I could come back and take the finals in six months or so when Katherine had stabilized.

My dad drove out to Malibu and met with the deans. "My son's life is never going to be the same. He's not going to be able to revisit these finals next fall, or ever. That season is over. You need to let him graduate. Figure out a way. Find a loophole. You're attorneys. It's what you do."

Amazingly, they figured out a way for me to graduate without taking finals but also without setting a negative precedent for the institution. As I walked across the stage erected on Pepperdine's grassy front lawn, the Pacific Ocean just behind me, I was reminded of God's undeniable provision in our life. Not just for the graduation, but for bringing us to this amazing place, to this community of wonderful people, and to such close proximity to the hospital that had saved Katherine's life.

As I received my diploma from our dean, Ken Starr, he hugged me tightly and whispered his heartfelt assurances that Katherine would be so proud, as the audience gave me a standing ovation. That afternoon, we delayed our return to the hospital for a bit and ate a weary but celebratory lunch at the Getty Villa Museum in Malibu, a special reservation Katherine had organized for my big day before her stroke. Though she was not there in person, the fingerprints of my biggest cheerleader were all over it.

Six weeks after the stroke, Katherine was weaned off the respirator that had breathed life into her lungs when she could not. She was now fully able to breathe on her own. This milestone was a miraculous answer to prayer, and it was the prerequisite for her to be able to leave the ICU and move on to a more therapy-focused phase of her recovery.

In counting back, I was shocked to discover she had been in the ICU for forty days. In the Bible, the number forty is used over and over again to signify periods of trial and testing. There was something indescribably hopeful in the notion that perhaps on the other end of this ICU wilderness period we might now be entering some kind of "promised land."

A few weeks before, her ventriculostomy tube had been removed from the top of her head, and amazingly, no permanent brain shunt was needed, as her brain could now regulate its own cerebrospinal fluid. Across the board, it was becoming clear that Katherine's body was able to recover; it just needed a long time to do so. Despite being freed from several machines, she was discharged from the ICU to a regular hospital bed, still bearing permanent IV ports and a trach and a G-tube and catheters. She hardly seemed well enough to leave, but the decision was made. We had been there longer than any patient we knew of.

As we left the ICU, we were surprised at the strange feeling of pining for a place that embodied the most horrific suffering of our lives. Perhaps it was not that different from the thought process of the freed Israelites who, as they wandered in the wilderness on their way to the Promised Land, still longed for the comfort and familiarity of their old lives of slavery in Egypt. For us, the ICU meant security and safety and privacy. There was always someone just a few steps away, day and night, monitoring Katherine, attending to her every need. The floor she went to had one nurse for eight patients, and we were assigned to a room shared with an older woman who had suffered a minor stroke and was also diabetic. I stayed with Katherine that first night, and neither of us slept a wink as our new roommate on the other side of the curtain divider had frantic blood sugar drops at all hours that required the noisy intervention of medical personnel. If only we could go back to the ICU where it was quiet. Funny how quickly we rewrite our painful pasts as a means to avoid the risky and unknown but ultimately life-giving future.

The next day, an empty room opened up next door into which we gladly and rapidly moved. We were exhausted after the hugely emotional transition and the sleepless night. I was also heavily burdened by the reality that I would need to decide where Katherine would go from here. We could stay on "The Floor" only until she got into a neurological acute rehabilitation unit where she would begin the next phase of her recovery. This would be the place where she would hopefully learn to sit up and walk and talk again. While there was one just a few floors below us at UCLA, it had only eleven beds, and we were cautioned to look at other options, as it was unlikely Katherine would be able to be admitted there.

I had dozed off next to Katherine's bedside and was awakened by a soft knock on our door. A man dressed in a suit walked into the room. He didn't appear to be a doctor, and I didn't recognize him, but his UCLA badge indicated he worked for the hospital in some official capacity. Without even formally introducing himself, he asked, "Jay, is there anything I can do to improve your stay here?" My mind was foggy from lack of sleep, but I was annoyed that the room's main overhead light was out. "I guess you can change that lightbulb if you want." He smiled.

I racked my brain to think of anything else but could not. He shook my hand warmly, gave me his business card, and proceeded to leave. Suddenly, I remembered and stammered out,

"Oh, you know, we're trying to figure out where Katherine can go to acute rehab. We would love to stay here at UCLA, but I know it's hard to get into that unit. Maybe you could help us." He nodded reassuringly and left.

I all but forgot about the strange visitor until I was awakened again by a call later that afternoon. "Mr. Wolf, I'm calling from UCLA's Neuro Rehab Unit. We have a bed available for Katherine. She can move down here tomorrow." I was so shocked that my prayers had been answered so quickly. This was the perfect next step for Katherine. UCLA had helped save her life and had helped stabilize her. Now, I knew they would help her get her life back.

Relief flooded through me, and I stared down at Katherine, feeling more hopeful than I had in a long time. I fished around in my pocket and grasped the business card of the stranger earlier in the day. I looked at it for the first time with a stupefied grin on my face. It read, "Dr. David Feinberg, CEO, UCLA Medical Center."

PART TWO

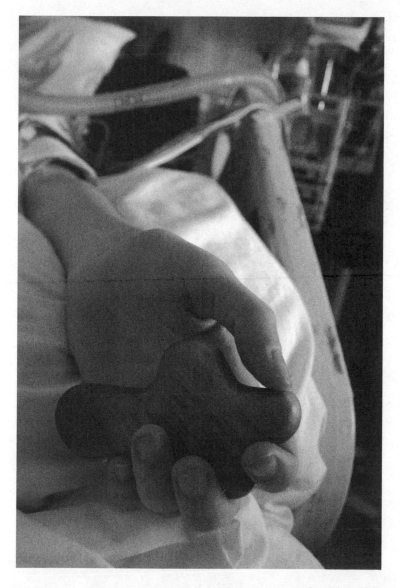

THE HOPE DEFERRED

Katherine

My eyes fluttered open, and I looked around the white room. It was like waking up from a dream, but all of a sudden the fog began to lift and the questions began to flood my mind. *Where am I? What has happened to me?*

I tried to call out to Jay, who was sitting in the corner, but my voice wouldn't make any noise. He saw that my eyes were open and came over to me with a concerned look as I started to become aware of the tubes coming from my arms and the strange pieces of plastic and rubber in my throat and in my upper abdomen. Jay patted me in the calming way he does, and I felt momentarily relieved somehow.

Besides a few flashes of the faces of family and friends in the ICU, I had no memories from the first two and a half months after the stroke. Apparently, I had been conscious and even interacting with people, but I couldn't remember any of it.

Suddenly, I nearly jumped out of bed as a thought rushed to my mind: *Where is my baby?!*

Before long, our dear friends Anna and Andy came in, carrying James in their arms. I later learned they were taking care of him so my family could focus on taking care of me. My mother's heart leapt to see James, my little sidekick. I didn't know how long it had been since I had seen him, but it surely could not have been more than a day or two. He seemed distant from me. I thought that surely my little guy hadn't forgotten me in only a couple of days.

Surely he must be hungry. We'll fix that right up. I figured I would feed him right then and there. *Come here, my baby.* I reached out my left arm to him, catching it on one of the tubes. My right arm did not seem to be lifting easily. *Maybe it's asleep.*

I quickly tried to figure out the logistics of how I could feed him. *Maybe the hospital bed will tilt, and I can sit up. But I don't know what to do about this big tube sticking out of my stomach just below my breast. Maybe we can take that out?*

Just as my plan was beginning to come together, James began to cry. Anna said it was his naptime. As she brought him close to say good-bye, I once again tried to lift my arms to hold him. *I can make him stop crying*, I thought, though no words would come out of my mouth. *I'm his mommy. I'm his mommy.* Then Anna took him out of the room.

Like a recurring bad dream, this same scene replayed every day. James would visit me, and my mind would race to figure out how to hold him and feed him. He needed me. I didn't know how he was getting fed. He was a breastfed baby; we had never even tried formula. *Somebody tell them that!*

I was exhausted in a way I had never been, much more than during the sleep-deprived months after James's birth. Every inch of my body felt heavier, like moving underwater, but my motherly instincts gave me just enough energy to focus obsessively on the one task of feeding my baby.

But one day after my visit with James, the reality hit me like a slap across the face: James had been fed and cared for by others for weeks now. It was suddenly so clear, and I began to weep silently. The truth hurt so much more than the IVs in my arm and the tubes in my throat and stomach.

I slowly began to understand that I had survived a brain bleed and that I was this "slow-motion miracle girl." I learned that I had been on life support for more than a month, and the professionals hadn't thought I would ever be able to downgrade from Intensive Care. I had defied all odds and was progressing more than anyone would have ever imagined I could.

I also eventually learned I could no longer walk, eat, hear

out of my right ear, see one image at a time, speak clearly, or use my right arm or hand. Hey, I was a big ole miracle, though. I guess that was a comfort to my friends and family. I felt no comfort at all. In fact, the whole miracle thing really stung because the "miracle" had left me unable to live normally.

I racked my brain for what I could have ever done to invoke such anger and wrath in a God who was clearly punishing me. Instead of a profound miracle of God, I saw this as a cruel curse straight from the pit of hell. *How can I live this way? I have a baby at home. I'm twenty-six years old. What does the future look like now?* The sadness was almost overwhelming. *Why me, God? Why not just go ahead and take me home to heaven?*

I had never felt more trapped and confused. Having always been an eternal optimist, I had never before known the terrifying feeling of losing the will to live.

Fortunately, the therapy life would not allow me to contemplate such feelings for long. I was thrust into a rigorous schedule of daily activities. Family and friends also filled my days and nights with scheduled shifts and sleepovers. It was almost too much to handle, but I began to recognize these routines as much-needed structure in the midst of my chaotic life reversal. If it had been up to me, I'm not sure I would have even desired to get out of bed in the morning, but none of my people were going to let me stay there. They were going to get me up and get me well again and get me back to my life with Jay and James. If *they* thought I could do it, I suppose *I* did too. After all, I wasn't doing it alone.

Fairly early in my new hospital room, I started to get powerful food cravings. I was being nourished by a high-calorie gray liquid poured through a tube directly into my stomach four to six times a day, and yet thoughts of food or beverage of any kind made my mouth water and sent me into an intense hyperfocus on eating and chewing and swallowing. I quickly learned I was "NPO" ("Nothing per Oral") and had been this way since the stroke/surgery. My swallowing nerves had been compromised—possibly beyond repair—in order to remove all of the AVM.

Every night, in the early evening, various relatives and friends would visit me, stay for a half hour or so, and then excuse themselves. I didn't think too much of it. After multiple weeks, I finally caught on to what was happening. There was a break room across the hall from my room, and all food was kept there. Family and friends would take turns eating in that room and being with me.

It hit me hard that I was *not* eating, while everyone around me *was* eating. They would never eat in front of me, but I had razor-sharp intuition about anyone eating anything at any time or any place. I felt so left out, like I was back in third grade and couldn't go to the cool kids' area of the playground at recess. But when I finally made the connection that these friends had signed up to bring a hot meal every night for my family, I was so touched by this sweet way our loving community was expressing support. Amazingly, this would continue throughout our entire stay at UCLA. They would drop off the meal, visit with me while my family ate in the break room, and then leave while my family stayed with me until bedtime.

Still, one day I had had it with this no-eating/hospital thing and decided to take matters into my own hands. My friend Suzanne had shown me pictures of her recent trip to Cabo San Lucas. That seemed like a good place to visit after I managed to get all the leftovers from my family's last meal. I was sure the leftovers from their dinner would include coconut cake, jelly-filled donuts, slabs of smoked salmon, dark chocolate caramels with sea salt, French press coffee, and Hot Tamales candies. Clearly, those were the foods in the break room. With a final destination in mind, all I needed to do now was to wait for the moment when I could sneak across the hall to get the free food and then continue to the airport. I would change out of my hospital gown in the airport bathroom. It was a plan! I could almost taste the yummy feast and feel the warm sand between my toes.

Once I thought the coast was clear, I sat up and got quickly out of bed. I hit the floor very hard. The friend who had been with me—but had left me for a moment to take a quick bathroom break—heard the thud and ran in, crying and screaming in horror. Alarms began to sound, and a nurse ran in to check me for injuries and resettle me back in bed. While I had no injuries from the fall—except for a very sad and confused heart—I knew there would be no leftovers and no trip to the beach. It was a slow and painful realization, but I eventually got the picture that I would not be leaving this room for a long, long time.

The Neuro Rehab Unit at UCLA was our new home. Thankfully, Katherine was once again in a private room where she could feel safe and able to get the rest she needed. Unlike the ICU, overnight visitors were allowed and even encouraged, and it seemed Katherine rested much better when she was not alone. I stayed most nights, but thankfully our friends stepped in and offered their overnight services, staying with Katherine so I could get better-quality sleep a few times a week. My father-in-law would always take the early morning shift when he was in town, arriving at 6:00 a.m. with hot coffee and his contagious positivity. We settled into this new routine, reenergized and yearning more deeply than ever for Katherine to progress in this next phase of recovery. It was a season of greater stability, but one with more emotional strain as the crisis-mode adrenaline began to fade and the reality of our situation began to sink in.

Though the hospital continued to be top-notch and all the medical professionals gave us excellent care, the weeks of hospital life had communicated something clearly to me: Doctors are only humans too. I realized that my role went beyond being Katherine's strong, silent supporter. I suppose the recent years of legal training I had just completed naturally led me to the role of being her advocate regarding medical, insurance, and even familial issues. Beside Katherine herself, I had the most to gain and the most to lose in the outcomes of her recovery, so I made it my mission to assure she was receiving the most diligent aid, that the right questions were being asked, and that the atmosphere surrounding her was one of peace and order.

Somehow, my natural bent toward details came into even greater focus despite emotional and physical fatigue, and I tried to hold the staff and our friends accountable to the highest standards of care without rudely overstepping my bounds. It was a challenging balance but a holy burden that I felt called to like no other calling in my life. Ironically, one of the main reasons I was able to fully live into this new role had to do with a game show.

Nearly a year earlier, we were in a coffee shop when Katherine was approached by a casting director for the television show "Are You Smarter Than a 5th Grader?" The show was looking for a pregnant contestant, and Katherine was offered a spot. After a few weeks of pondering whether or not she could handle the potential humiliation of her bloopers posted on YouTube for all the world to see, Katherine bravely decided to dust off her elementary school flash cards and go for it. Hilariously and providentially, she correctly answered only three out of six fifth-grade-level trivia questions (the other three were answered by actual fifth graders, thus saving her from elimination), but nonetheless, she won $50,000! Of course, the fine print in the contract said there would be no actual winnings unless her show aired. Thankfully, in April 2008, just weeks before the stroke, her episode did air, and I got the check in the mail the first week she was in acute rehab. That unexpected gift enabled me to do what many loved ones are unable to do: focus on being a full-time caregiver. It was a clear sign that God would provide a way for our family to survive this tragedy together. He would work in the mundane and in the extraordinary, and He would use our families and church community, a game show, and anything in between to do it.

We were getting used to these new routines and new faces, new regulations and new prognoses. Katherine had been awake and responsive since the first day after her surgery, but it was growing more and more apparent that she had not really been fully awake at all. The fact that she was beginning to process her injury more fully was a painful revelation. Her previously calm, almost saint-like behavior in the ICU had inspired us as we grappled to find peace in the midst of this storm. We had naively hoped that Katherine had somehow magically bypassed the normal human stages of grief and had arrived at some transcendent peace about her situation right out of the gate. In reality, three months after her stroke, she was only just beginning to be aware of all she had lost.

One Friday night within the first few weeks of our arrival in acute rehab, we decided to pretend we were having a normal, relaxing evening together, watching TV in bed. I hadn't gotten all the way in bed with Katherine until then, as I was concerned about sitting on a catheter or pulling out an IV needle, or knocking off the respirator tube. Yet I knew the value of human touch and connection for Katherine. When she motioned to me to lie beside her, I smiled, letting down my guard.

Her bed was equipped with an air mattress to help prevent bedsores, and as I squeezed myself next to her between the bedrails, the mattress squished awkwardly. I shifted my weight one way and then another, only exacerbating the situation. Our sweet attempt at a "normal date night" suddenly morphed into something altogether different as Katherine unexpectedly lurched upright and began to manically push me away. It was as if her change in position on the bed suddenly changed her emotional state as well. She began to weep, a terrifying soundless cry. She tore at her IVs and her breathing tube in claustrophobic and agitated fury, like a caged animal. Her tracheostomy began to bleed.

I jumped up in horror at the fire I had inadvertently lit inside her. She seemed like a different person—no longer the ethereal, angelic patient we had been seeing. It was as if in a moment, the frustration, the pain, and the fear of her new world collapsed on top of her, and she was violently struggling to claw her way out.

Her nurse came in and fixed her back up. She finally calmed down and soon exhaustedly fell asleep. I slipped into the bathroom and began to cry hard, both for the pain I had accidentally elicited in her and for the fear that all this pain was changing her at her very core into someone and something altogether different.

However, the location of her AVM in her cerebellum led the medical staff to believe that, although her physical and motor deficits were great, there was little to no cognitive deficit. Unlike an injury to the frontal lobe of the brain, Katherine's memories, personality, and language would be unaffected. This was such a vital, hopeful component to her impossibly painful circumstances. The only thing worse than having your body stripped of its ability to function is having your brain stripped of its ability to function too. In those cases, recovery is so much harder because there may be no will to fight, no memories to inspire hope, no ability to regain purpose, no faith to fuel perseverance.

At the same time, we were now confronted with the reality of a patient coming alive again—alive to a different body and a different world. She was in there, and she was in pain, and I could not fix it.

After weeks of staying at a church friend's rather spectacular bachelor pad near the hospital, it was evident to me that we would not be going home anytime soon. Despite the generous hospitality, I needed a place of our own to stay. All our things remained at the married housing apartment on Pepperdine's campus, the one we had called our first home as a married couple, the place we brought James home to from the hospital. Because Malibu is nearly an hour away from the UCLA Medical Center, I had returned to the apartment only a couple times.

As a new wave of students would be descending on the campus in the coming weeks and months, I needed to move out. Despite offers of help, I decided to go alone. Our lives had been unwillingly dismantled by the stroke, and I wanted to be the one to gently gather the pieces and pack them up so they might be reassembled into a new life and a new home someday.

Entering the apartment was like stepping into a still-life portrait. The apartment was just as it had been left on April 21, save for a much-appreciated cleaning of Katherine's vomit off the rug and a general straightening up of the place by our law school friends, including throwing away the two lasagnas Katherine was in the middle of making as her brain began to hemorrhage. Weeks after this, one of the first things she would ask me when she could speak again was, "What did you do with the lasagnas? Did you put them in the fridge? I hope you saved them." I think I just nodded.

Sadly, the remnants of her love-made-edible were long gone, but their memory and the memories of so many moments of our early adult life lingered there. Flashes of a life we had come to love included many memories at the table. Like the time we hosted all the stragglers for Thanksgiving, cobbling together chairs and uneven tabletops into one long communal gathering, passing around homemade recipes gathered from Southern grandmas and then walking it all off, barefoot, on the beach that night as the sun set. Or the time when we invited Dr. Phillips, whom I credit with helping me get into law school, for dinner and served him nearly raw steak and soupy chocolate pecan pie, and he ate every bite with a gentlemanly exuberance that extinguished some of our own silent horror at our unrefined cooking skills. Or the time when we spread blankets on the living room rug for an impromptu Parisian-inspired picnic for Valentine's Day two months before the stroke, breaking baguettes smeared with soft cheese in flickering candlelight while James cooed in his bouncy seat next to us.

In the quiet, sometimes the voices finally stop; but sometimes the deepest ones finally begin to speak. I wandered through each of the rooms in that place, touching the walls and the tops of the furniture, opening the closets and stepping into Katherine's smells, breathing in the essence of a much-loved life, nearly choking on its sweetness. *What are we going to do? What are we going to do?* The soul-pain welled up, throbbing, stinging, heart strangling. I felt the pain for myself, but more so for Katherine. I resolved that since Katherine would get no good-byes to the life that was ripped from her, I must say them for her.

I began to clean and straighten the apartment like I never had before, creating the best version of it—perhaps a never-before-realized version, given the constraints of grad school and new parenthood. When I was finished, I took out my camera and begin to photograph each room, precariously balancing on chairs and ledges to get the best angles, shooting pictures in memoriam until the late afternoon light turned to dusk. These would be Katherine's good-byes.

The campus bells tolled in the distance, a kind of requiem

for the death of this place and the happy lives lived here. I sat staring out across the parking lot, straining for a last glimpse at the smear of blue ocean in the distance before dusk turned to night. And then it was finished, not because I wanted it to be, but because the time had come, the light had gone, and there was much to do before morning.

James, my sister Sarah, and I moved into a new apartment near the hospital that week. It had never been lived in before and had marble countertops and red-tiled rooftops and courtyards with splashing fountains. It was shiny and new, but also characterless and cookie-cutter. Nevertheless, perhaps it was a blank slate on which to create a new story of us.

On Saturdays, a recreational therapist would sometimes come to acute rehab to engage patients in nonhospital experiences. Since Katherine had only seen the last of our Pepperdine apartment through my photographs, I wanted her to see this new home, maybe the place she would soon call home too. The therapist lovingly accepted my proposed form of recreational therapy and wheeled Katherine the three blocks from her hospital room to the new apartment, likely breaking some liability protocol. In so doing, he was giving Katherine something far wilder and riskier than a simple trip outside of the hospital confines; he was giving her hope.

It was her first time being rolled down normal sidewalks, past joggers and commuters, dappled sunlight kissing her hospital-white arms. It felt like we were nonchalantly smuggling a priceless sculpture out of a museum, having donned said sculpture with a floppy hat and tourist sunglasses, plopping it in a wheelchair, covering it with a blanket, and whistling inconspicuously, "Oh, nothing to see here, officer."

We arrived at the apartment, and her eyes lit up as they had when James visited her bedside, and her half-paralyzed mouth excitedly formed dramatic oohs and aahs. We helped her out of her chair and onto the balcony. On the sidewalk below, her unsuspecting mom was walking with groceries and nearly had a heart attack at the sight of her hospital-bound daughter excitedly waving from above.

This could be home. Katherine could come home again.

Katherine

I had not seen myself in a mirror yet. It just hadn't been a priority to anyone. Since "waking up," I had hardly thought about my appearance in light of more pressing issues related to my new disabled condition.

I could feel (or not feel, I guess) that the right side of my face was totally numb. In fact, it felt as though a line had been drawn from my forehead to my chin, straight down the middle. There was completely normal feeling on the left, zero feeling on the right. However, the thought had never entered my mind that numbness could equal paralysis. I assumed all the sad faces upon observing me were about the situation I was in, not my appearance.

Once I gained access to a mirror, I just stared and stared in disbelief. It was shocking. *Why won't my face move on the right side? Why didn't anyone tell me? Why didn't anyone warn me?*

By far the worst realization was that I now had an eye facing downward and quirking to the right, looking toward my nose. It was appalling. I could see out of it, but my vision had been very blurry since the stroke. I was also seeing double of everything, which was maddening and disorienting. Also, I didn't realize that while I was in the ICU, my right eye couldn't fully shut, and it didn't blink automatically throughout the day. As a result, my eye got completely dried out, and my cornea was torn. It had improved some, but it still didn't lubricate itself properly.

Since I hadn't been in direct sunlight in more than two months, my hair had started to turn a brownish-gray color that aged me tremendously. I am already fair-skinned, but now I looked ghostly white, except for big black circles under my eyes. I had lost almost twenty-five pounds, and this made me bony and angular. My face looked sharp and jagged and intense. I appeared gaunt and exhausted.

I was horrified by the ghastly look of frailty and death. I was beyond sad. I never thought I was overly focused on my appearance, not any more than your typical Southern gal. But this was shocking. Not only did I not feel beautiful; I didn't even recognize myself. Yet as hard as it was to look in the mirror, it was harder to not look. I needed to see this new me. I needed to know what I was up against. I needed to understand the reality so I could focus on getting well again and returning to life with Jay and James. Theirs were the only opinions that really mattered, and each time James nuzzled up to me in the hospital bed or Jay looked at me lovingly, I knew my two guys would always think I was beautiful anyway.

After more weeks of coming to/waking up, I started to understand that half of my care team was comprised of male nurses. The various men were deeply respectful and took excellent care of me the entire time I was under their world-class treatment. Surely, much of my recovery could be attributed to their expertise and meticulous concern for my many issues.

With that said, my thoughts during that time were jumbled and disturbing. *Why is that man changing my hospital gown? Why is he giving me a sponge bath? Is he going to molest me or rape me? Can I trust him? Why is he here? GO AWAY! LEAVE*

*ME ALONE! DON'T TOUCH ME! I don't need a bath. You
just want to see me naked, you perverts! GET OUT OF MY
ROOM!* Since I could not speak and did not want to hurt their
feelings, I didn't utter a sound as I silently and reluctantly complied with their care.

In my more lucid moments, I felt ashamed by my thoughts
toward these sweet men who were trying to make me well, but
I was also petrified at being so weak and vulnerable and easily
taken advantage of. My body was totally powerless, and it was
a horrible feeling.

Over time, I got more used to this bizarre new world of
immodesty and indignities. *They are helping me. They are here
so I can get well and go home. They are like brothers.* But they
weren't my brothers. They were grown men with wives and
children and lives and stories and mothers and grandmothers.
I wanted to respect their families, especially their wives. *These
married men should not see other women naked. It's just not
right. Is it?*

I tried to adjust, but there were several areas of care that
were off-limits to anyone except family. While I had a urinary
catheter and felt perfectly fine about men or women changing it
out, when I needed a bedpan, I would wait for my mom or one
of my sisters. Getting on and off a bedpan was very difficult
for a person lacking balance and coordination. The females in
my family would help make that process more bearable—and
sometimes even funny for me.

My mom and sisters understood my feelings toward male
nurses and the awkwardness of sponge bathing in general, so
they started giving me yummy-smelling sponge baths and washing my hair every Sunday. A good shampooing and blow-dry
would leave me feeling like a new woman. Once, my mom even
managed to get a drugstore "cap" and weave highlights into
my mousy brown hair. One sister would paint my toenails and
shave my legs; the other would paint my fingernails and shave

my armpits. Our spa days were dignifying and thus glorious for me, and they became the highlight of my week. While I yearned for some edible spa treats too, even just a cucumber water, the tender care offered by women who loved me satisfied a deep need in my soul. While our relationships with each other were just as imperfect as in any other family, those Sundays together were a carefree time of much more than beauty treatments; they were a cathartic cry of "we've still got it!" We could have fun together, despite this nightmare.

Because of my tracheostomy, the air was escaping prior to reaching my mouth so I could not manufacture sounds. Also, I was so exhausted and weak that I didn't have the energy to push out words. Much to my delight, I was given a letter board. This small device allowed me to type a letter, and then the small computer would speak the letter. I could use my working left hand and hit the keys to make words. The letter board provided an ability to communicate without worrying about trying to speak with no sound coming out.

I would mostly use the letter board to communicate when my expressive nonverbals wouldn't cut it. Much of the time, the board was not necessary, since I could use my facial expressions or could mouth words, but it was very useful for "saying" something that no one could get but that I *needed* them to get.

I would also frequently use it for non sequiturs (which I'm famous for using). Often, I would punch out J A M E S just so somebody would start to talk about that little cutie I missed so badly. The board became this strange conversation-changing device. It was almost fun. Almost.

When I had deep truths to communicate, I would use the board as well. I typed over and over, *I'm the same on the inside! I'm the same on the inside!* because I wanted everyone to know that. While I was messed up on the outside, most of the rehab patients around me were messed up on the inside. I still had my memories, my personality, my faith. Even though my appearance and bodily functions had changed, that is where it stopped. I was more motivated to convey that everything was the same internally than any other "words" I needed "spoken" by Mr. Board Man. I wanted my family, friends, nurses, therapists, candy stripers, janitors, etc. to know that I might look totally different, but nothing had changed inside me. *What if they don't understand that? What if everyone thinks I've got the IQ of a small child now or no memory at all? What if I'm deemed an unfit mother for James? What if no one knows that cognitively I'm exactly the same as I was on April 20, 2008?* I was horrified at the thought that people wouldn't realize I was still "all there." Unanswered questions tormented me in my silence.

Yet I felt a deep comfort that God would help me in this terrible situation. He knew I was in this broken "earth suit" and couldn't fully communicate my heart to anyone. I felt a deep comfort that He would make it okay. He would handle it. I just needed to be still and wait.

Katherine began therapy for her speech and her swallowing early in her stay in acute rehab. As much as she wanted to stand and walk and use her right hand, her inability to talk and eat hit at the crux of her identity. Her patience in waiting for their return was fading quickly.

The nerves that control the complex swallowing movement were compromised to an uncertain degree during her life-saving brain surgery. I learned that this network of intracranial nerves sprouting from the brain stem to vital areas of the head and neck are as thin as hairs and the consistency of butter, making it difficult to know the exact effect of any trauma to them. While there was great hope in the plasticity of the brain and rewiring of the neural pathways, there was almost no hope in the regrowth of these specific types of nerves once they'd been damaged. Though her right side from head to toe was greatly impaired, Katherine retained fairly normal function on the left side of her face and body, including her mouth and down her throat, so it seemed possible that some sort of speech and swallowing might occur with enough practice.

For weeks, Katherine engaged in the most basic speech therapies, first learning how to move her partially paralyzed tongue and form her left-leaning lips into different shapes. She continued to use her letter board, though precise spelling was complicated due to her double vision. All of these once-effortless actions now felt impossibly challenging. Their surprising complexity frustrated Katherine but motivated her all the more to press on toward the goal of speaking and swallowing normally again.

After weeks of practice, Katherine's speech therapist decided it was time for some vocalization. There had been much anticipation, and now a sense of relief, for us all that Katherine would be able to communicate again with her words. Not being able to express herself effectively had been a huge hardship, especially for one who had always been a "Chatty Cathy." Even as a young child, Katherine had already used her verbal capacities more than most men do in a lifetime. At the age of two, she would pepper her even-tempered dad with so many questions that he would have to ask her to please take a little break from talking. Her gift of gab only increased through the years, from endless theatre productions to majoring in communication studies in college. We all knew Katherine had so much more to say than her left hand, left eye, and left finger typing on the letter board could adequately convey. What would she say first? Would she talk for three months straight to make up for the three months of silence?

Though she no longer needed help breathing, her breathing tube would not be removed until it was absolutely confirmed that she could fully oxygenate her blood on her own. In order to regain her voice, the trach had to be capped so the air forced up through her lungs could pass over her vocal cords rather than escape out of the trach hole. As the speech therapist placed the Passy-Muir speaking valve on the hole of the trach, I waited for some sort of wafting essence to suddenly swirl up around her body and for her voice to come bursting out, strong and crystal clear. Of course, three months of nonuse had taken its toll, and the thing that had once drawn me to Katherine—the singsong, rapid-fire, confident quality in her ability to communicate with her words—was gone. As though she had consumed a glassful of dust, her first wispy strains of rebirthed speech rasped weakly, creating nothing but an inharmonious sound. Nevertheless, the therapist wasted no time instructing Katherine how to take this new voice for a ride.

Soon, she began to form out of this dust real, living words. With an unusual symphonic quality, like a rarely used fireplace bellow, she wheezed out "hello" and then "blue." Her voice was much lower than normal and sounded so unfamiliar. The instant she spoke these childlike words into the world—words that James would soon be learning for the first time too—I began to weep. This was not the voice I had known or the voice I had expected to hear that day. But it was a voice born through dust and ashes—the voice of a soul straining for new life—and it was breathtakingly beautiful to me. Equipped with a new voice and filled with questions in need of answers, Katherine began to come to life again. After all, this was a speech therapy victory, so her focus shifted to similar victories in her swallow therapy. Despite the charm of her simple new vocabulary, with phrases like "hi, how are ya?" greeting everyone she encountered, she began to lose some of her Southern belle gentility, becoming incredulous as to why her swallowing therapist would not even let her drink a little water or crunch an ice cube. She began to focus on this obsessively in the same way a thirsty traveler lost in the desert might become unhinged looking for water.

As I observed and compared this situation to advice we were receiving from other medical professionals we had contacted across the country, it became clear that in the swallowing therapy world, there were different schools of thought. It seemed that UCLA subscribed to the more conservative, "old school" variety. Katherine was not allowed to even have liquid in her mouth because there was a fear that the water could easily trickle down into her lungs and cause pneumonia, which could be life-threatening, as she was still immobile.

Emboldened by Katherine's improving speech, I approached the lead swallowing therapist in my role as medical advocate, hoping I might be able to convince her to try some new techniques. Equipped with some research I had done on other methods of swallow therapy that she could employ, I knocked on her door confidently. She invited me to come into her office, just down the hall from Katherine's room. I didn't know her well, so I began to ask her some questions about herself and quickly ascertained that she was a caregiver for her husband, who had been sick for a long time. Without knowing the full scope of his ailment or their history, it became clear that her life was full of more pain and disappointments than her professional demeanor would let on. She quickly shifted topics and cut to the chase before I had time to segue into my enlightening research. "Mr. Wolf, you need to understand that I cannot give Katherine water—or anything, for that matter—because she cannot swallow. Honestly, given the severe damage to her swallowing nerves, it is unlikely she will ever be able to swallow again."

The shocking severity of this statement must have clicked

off my attention for a moment because the next thing I remember hearing was, "Do you understand what I'm saying to you? Katherine will likely never eat again. You need to prepare yourself and her for this reality."

I excused myself and exited quickly, feeling a sense of disbelief and rage welling up inside me. In my entire life I had never heard of a person not being able to eat. I took a deep breath, trying to exhale out the despair I felt settling in. For Katherine and me, eating was not just some means to an end; we lived to eat. We even met in the cafeteria! What a cruel irony; what a tasteless joke! Of all the functions a body could lose, why this one?

I didn't know the therapist's motivation in casting this horrific prophecy over Katherine's recovery. Maybe her husband could not eat either, and she didn't want me to get my hopes up; or maybe she resented the expectant, starry-eyed spirit that Katherine's story brought to the rehab unit. Regardless of whether or not I fully believed her words, I never forgot them. They served as a warning but also as a challenge. Yet I knew this horrible prognosis would bring no momentum to Katherine's tremendous uphill efforts to relearn to speak and swallow and live again. Those simple words—"Katherine will likely never eat again"—might be the first domino knocked over, setting off a chain reaction, taking down every last one of us into a morass of hopelessness. Though Katherine and I had always shared everything, I vowed to never tell her what the therapist said, at least not until she proved everybody wrong.

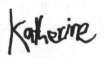

"I'm hangry!" This is a combination of the words *hungry* and *angry,* and it sadly became one of the most appropriate descriptions of the not-eating part of my life. Just months before, I had

been on a "take no prisoners" pregnancy binge, eating whatever might make me not feel nauseous, which usually involved
fried carbs or chocolate. Then most recently, post-pregnancy
breastfeeding and sleepless nights had elicited a different manic
craving for calories and life-sustaining hot coffee. Now, while I
could almost taste and smell those imaginary feasts, that was all
they were: imaginary. I recalled a story describing heaven and
hell as feasts where a person could eat only with a very long-
handled spoon. In hell, everyone unsuccessfully tried to feed
themselves, while in heaven, they fed each other. Since I could
not feed myself, nor would anyone else feed me, where exactly
did that leave me?

I had heard stories of NPO patients being given ice chips.
These could satisfy the tongue with the cold stimulation, and
the melted water would not greatly affect the lungs in case of
aspiration. I became obsessed with ice chips. My mouth began
to burn, and I knew it was at least two hundred degrees in there.
I needed ice chips to bring down the temperature in my mouth.
None were given, despite my daily requests. I even tried to bribe
my speech therapist for some "under the table" chips at one
point. I told her I had access to large amounts of cash; the cash
was hers in exchange for ice chips. I was that desperate and
delirious. The therapist resisted the bribe and continued her
work of pushing on the back of my tongue with various long
Q-tips to try to initiate my swallow reflex. That was my first
and last attempt at bribing my therapists.

My cravings continued to be horrible. I was dying to have a
bowl of cereal, pancakes, or eggs for breakfast; a whole cookie
cake for dessert; and a gallon of hot coffee with hazelnut-flavored
creamer. I would have killed for a grilled cheese sandwich for
lunch, with a huge lemon bar for dessert, washed down with a
gallon of sweet tea; pasta for dinner with a meaty tomato sauce;
and Girl Scouts Thin Mints cookies for dessert with a glassful
of eggnog!

My speech therapist friend Leah came from out of town to lend her skills. In my most scandalous sleepover of all time, she barricaded the door and finally fed me those coveted ice chips. I kid you not, I felt as though I had been transported to a magical chocolate factory and had indulged in a decadent treat no one else on earth had tasted. It was euphoric. And true to what Leah already knew from her studies and experience, I could handle the ice chips just fine; and even if I didn't, it would still be fine. I did not so much as cough that night.

I knew that if I wanted to swallow normally, I would need to get the trach removed. It was as simple as that in my mind. Whenever the head nurse would come by my room to test if my blood oxygen level was stable enough for removal, I would try to breathe in a certain manner to get specific number reads on the pulse oximeter. Always unsuccessful, I was determined to get that number to match what she needed to see, because then I'd be able to get the trach out and be chowing down. One day, my breathing techniques actually worked. The trach was removed, and victory was mine! I knew I'd be eating just as soon as a doctor could sign off on a complete swallow reflex. The feeding tube would come out a few weeks after that, and getting real food in my system just *had* to aid in the recovery process. Eating *would* make me well again. And certainly my walking would kick in once I was able to start nourishing my body. This was the beginning of getting back on my feet. I was sure of it.

For my first official swallow test, I was taken to a doctor's office across the street from the hospital. My dad and Jay accompanied me as a nurse pushed the wheelchair. In the waiting room, I daydreamed about the first food I would consume. *Coconut cream pie or dark chocolate molten lava cake?* It was a hard decision. *Perhaps my swallow will still be fragile. Then I will do a milkshake! That will be so tasty and satisfying.* It was all settled in my mind by the time my name was called.

In the exam room, the doctor threaded a thin tube with a camera on the end into my right nostril and down my throat. The inside of my throat was projected in a disturbingly large version on a TV behind me. Then I was fed a green pudding and asked to swallow it as hard as I could. *Victory!* I cheered internally. But my crooked smile faded as the doctor asked, "Do you think you are actually swallowing?" Though it seemed to me I was swallowing normally, I was actually not swallowing at all, not even a little. The pudding just sat precariously in the back of my throat until the doctor scooped it out. My next memory is of my dad crying. I have seen my dad cry on only two other occasions in my entire life.

Everyone shared my grief over not being able to swallow because we all knew that eating is about so much more than food consumption. Eating is life! Eating is what humans do; it is how we socialize. If you cannot eat, you are in a weird world, all alone. You miss out on that natural sense of connection to people over a meal or a cup of coffee. It is very isolating because you are no longer a participant in normal life; you are watching life—a spectator. Not being able to eat or drink made me feel like a crazy person. I honestly thought that if I had to choose, I would rather never walk again than never eat again!

Because I had spent two months in a hospital bed, my body had changed drastically. Not only was I severely underweight, but I had also lost almost all of my muscle tone. My circulatory system was a wreck. Sitting up in bed caused me a type of dizziness I had never known before, because even this simple change in position caused my blood pressure to plummet.

Physical therapists began trying to get me to sit up in bed for longer periods of time. First, I would sit up for two minutes and then slowly work up to five and then eight and then ten.

Once I could sit up for fifteen minutes straight, the therapists were willing to try helping me stand up in a standing frame. A standing frame is a large device that would help me actually stand up without having to balance my own weight. I was put in Mr. Standing Frame, and he did the work for me! He helped me have the feeling of standing up again without having to worry about gravity dropping me straight to the ground.

After many more weeks, we began the process of relearning to walk. Several of the other rehab patients had been injured in motorcycle accidents, so in their honor, I named my half-paralyzed right leg "Harley" and my left leg "Davidson." The name of the game was to get Harley to take weight once again. Many of my walking problems had to do with the fact that Harley would not support any weight.

It would take three therapists holding me up, but I did begin to take steps forward again. We would "walk"/hobble through any and every hallway of that hospital we saw. Someone would walk behind us (usually Jay or my mom) and push my wheelchair so I could take frequent breaks to sit down. I especially liked walking by nurses' stations because I would get to encourage them. I had long loved the idea of encouraging the encouragers, and this was that principle at work. I knew my sad situation could have a deep impact on these professionals as they watched me relearn to do something so basic, which no one thought I would ever do again.

This experience made me look outside of myself, and in so doing, the excruciatingly slow and exhausting process of relearning to walk became more bearable. "I'm learning to walk again," I would tell any nurse with whom I made eye contact. "I should not ever get to do this. I almost died. Tell your patients anything is possible. Never give up hope."

Many nurses would choke up on the spot. I felt deeply comforted in knowing that my learning to walk again had that effect on them. I knew they had seen it all, and it would take something very inspirational to move them. I was struck by the surprising thought, *I could inspire people.* I did not know anything about websites or all the people worldwide who were following my story. I did know that these nurses were inspired. *I could be an inspiration.* It felt good. I was actually a word picture of broken things made new. I embodied hope. Not just for the patients they could tell about me, but in their own lives. My relearning to walk was this beautiful picture of healing. Even though I initially fought against this new calling of mine—this miracle girl's inspiring others from her wheelchair—I knew deep down that it was undeniable.

In addition to walking and using the standing frame, I would spend my physical therapy hours trying to strengthen my body and coordinate movements. As time went on, the careful therapists would help me to the ground, and I would get on all fours. From there, we would practice simply staying in that position for up to five minutes. That eventually became ten minutes, and then they would have me reach for objects while balancing on one arm. Ultimately, I would work up to planking. Strengthening my core was imperative. In fact, strengthening every part of my body was a must if I ever wanted to walk by myself again.

The routinized weeks in acute rehab turned that gorgeous Los Angeles summer into a revolving door of monotonous white-walled therapy sessions with only incremental improvements in Katherine's recovery to show for our white-knuckled efforts. To think that while in ICU I had believed, really believed, that she and I would be in my best man's wedding in a few weeks seemed laughable and pitiful. Even the normally sweet moments of engaging James became glaring reminders of this new reality, this life without the mommy and wife we had known. So it was often just easier to focus on the next mini-emergency, the next therapy session, or the next insurance-related question. Nonetheless, I felt purposeful and useful in the role I was playing for Katherine. I felt neither self-pitying nor self-congratulatory at my decision to focus on the daily recovery of my brain-injured wife. To me, this was not valiant martyrdom or selfless heroism; it was just what I needed to do, what I had promised to do, for the person I loved most in the world.

The head nurse of the rehab unit was a total character—a champion bowler and a mad-scientist type with wild hair and a booming laugh. She was a kind engager of our story, but she had been around and had seen it all in her years of rehab work. "You should know that couples under thirty who suffer a brain injury divorce at a rate of 90 percent." *Oh, thanks for that pep talk*, I thought.

"I tell you this because your high level of involvement in your wife's recovery puts you in a much greater likelihood of physical burnout and emotional breakdown."

Again, thanks for the pep talk! I understood what she was saying, but I felt undeterred from continuing in the way I was engaging Katherine's new life and recovery. I had been given the great gift of a family and a community that were supporting me undyingly. I had also been given the financial resources, like the game show winnings, to free me up from some of the monetary pressures that add insult to injury in medical crises. I had been raised in a family of all sisters and a pastor-father, making me no stranger to all things female or ministry related. These combined factors empowered me to keep on serving, loving, and walking through this suffering with Katherine, side by side and not as a distant, detached observer. I could not imagine the choices and sacrifices other grieving spouses had to make in order to keep their jobs and save their families by leaving their patient, but that was not my story, at least not now, so I whole-heartedly embraced the opportunity I had been given.

Seeing that her previous statistics had not been very motivating in altering my behavior, the head nurse approached my dad. "Your son is going to burn out if he keeps up this pace here. You really ought to encourage him to take a break." My dad appreciated her concern, and as any parent would do, he presented me with this information and lovingly offered me his aid.

"Why don't you take a break?" he asked. "Just a few days. We could drive you up to Yosemite, breathe in some fresh air, do some hiking, and you could clear your head a bit."

It was strange. The prospect of a few days of rejuvenation in the gorgeous wilds of Northern California should have excited me; after all, I felt as if I had hardly seen the sun in months, and I was so tired of breathing in hospital air and hiking hospital halls. Yet for some reason, the prospect of leaving Katherine and my new assignment was entirely unappealing.

"Dad, Katherine can't take a vacation from all of this, so I'm not going to either. Thanks for the offer, but I'll wait to go to Yosemite when she and James can go with me."

My dad smiled knowingly and gave me a big hug. Later that day, he confidently reported back to the head nurse. "My son is going to keep coming here every day, and we are all going to support him as he supports Katherine. And you know what? I think they are both going to be just fine."

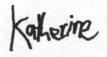

Several weeks into my ordeal, my family requested a meeting with Dr. Gonzalez, to review what had actually happened to me and to discuss what to expect from that point on. It is not uncommon for the patient and family to not know exactly what transpired during a crisis because it just isn't possible to absorb all the information at the time of the trauma and its aftermath.

When Dr. Gonzalez came to my hospital room to fill us in on the details, I still was not prepared for what would come out of his mouth. The full reality of what had happened stunned me.

"So I should have died," I said.

"No," he replied. "If you should have, then you would have."

I knew that "sacrifices" had been made to keep me alive. I knew that nerves had been damaged, and a sizable chunk of my cerebellum had been removed. The neurosurgeon had made it clear that day that my facial paralysis would be permanent. Those nerves were severed, and no therapy could salvage them. Ever.

Even though I was deeply disappointed, my hope soared when the doctor explained that the nerves affecting my swallowing had not been cut. In addition, he said that the brain could create new neural pathways to compensate for functions that had been lost, such as walking. I took that to mean my brain could make a comeback! I'm sure the doctor did not want to give me false hope; however, by saying that *anything* was not permanent, he gave me tremendous resolve. Now I was determined. I would defeat these pesky "deficits" because that was all they were—current deficits.

That is when my brain/nerve obsession began. Before that day, I knew nothing about the body's nerves or my own brain at all. Why would I? I was a young woman without a medical issue in the world. But armed with new knowledge, I was ready to take on the world. I just had to rehab like crazy and pray like crazy, and I would be eating again while skipping into my favorite restaurant.

Dr. Gonzalez recounted that he had recently presented my case to a group of UCLA doctors as a teaching case study. He showed my CT scans and reported my stats from the day in the emergency room and then asked his neurosurgery colleagues if they would have proceeded with the surgery. Not one of them said they would have chosen to do the surgery because of its complexity and my near-death condition.

The mood was somber because of the bleak prognosis for this anonymous patient, but when Dr. Gonzalez finished the presentation by explaining that not only did I survive the surgery, but I had also recovered so well that I was now in neuro rehab, his colleagues erupted into spontaneous applause.

While the slow pace of my recovery was terribly disheartening, we were encouraged by what we heard from Dr. Gonzalez. No matter what hard days lay ahead, undoubtedly the hardest one was over. The simple truth was that I should not be here, so the biggest victory had already been won. Surely the God who had conquered death was the same God who would continue to restore me back to life.

Katherine continued an excruciatingly slow recovery, but a recovery nonetheless. In time it became clear that, as in the ICU, we would soon hear the words, "You don't have to go home, but you can't stay here." We avoided the unit's social worker as one would a disgruntled boss. She had mentioned that our insurance was running out for this particular type of acute rehab medical benefit, a notion that was both maddening and relieving in a way. There would be an end to this monotonous, painstaking life of therapy, whether or not we wanted it to end. Regardless of the eventual outcomes in Katherine's recovery, there would be an end. And yet, as in the ICU, it was strangely hard to consider moving away from the safety and relative comfort of our current routine. Even though staying would likely mean plateauing and stagnation, it almost seemed worth it just to avoid another major change.

The social worker cornered me in the hallway. "Mr. Wolf, we need to discuss Katherine's next steps for recovery after her time here ends." She detailed our options, which boiled down to taking Katherine home or going to a long-term rehab facility. She recommended Casa Colina in Pomona, California, about an hour east of Los Angeles, yet so far outside of our LA bubble that it might as well have been on the East Coast. I wanted a third option, or at the very least I wanted someone to just tell me, based on all the factors in our lives, what we should do. Having already stood at more medical life-and-death crossroads for my family than most do in a lifetime, I was coming to the end of my decision-making rope.

Much to my frustration, none of the rehabbers wanted to box us in with their clinical opinions or even friendly advice as to what we should do next. It was clear that Katherine needed much, much more therapy, but it was extremely enticing to consider taking her home to the new apartment, comfortingly close to the hospital yet far away from these confining four walls. To get her and all of us out of this sterile setting and back into a home environment seemed logical, even obvious from an emotional standpoint. The social worker said insurance would even pay to bring therapists into our home a few times a week. I could envision this new life, all three of us playing house again until Katherine recovered more fully. And yet even these romanticized imaginings of a new life for our family couldn't eliminate the increasingly obvious elephant in the room: Katherine was still very, very sick.

It had been discussed that we might move back to the South to be near our families as Katherine entered a new phase of stability and recovery. Yet neither of us felt like it was the right move. We wanted to stay connected to the UCLA Medical Center and to our LA church community. It felt like the multifaceted purposes for our lives in Los Angeles had not yet come to an end.

In the discussions about Katherine's future recovery, we had encountered some "friend of friend" types—medical and rehab professionals, including one who actually owned an in-home rehab company in Southern California, the kind we would employ if we chose to move Katherine home. She had come to evaluate Katherine in the hospital a few days before. As I wrestled for informed wisdom, I asked her the golden question, "What would you do if this was your daughter?" With surprising candor and confidence, she answered, "If Katherine was my daughter, I would give her every chance at recovery I could by admitting her into a long-term rehab place. Casa Colina is one of the best neuro rehabs in the country. I would send her there."

It was the honesty I had longed for but the answer I had hoped not to hear. Yet, deep down, I think it was the decision I knew we needed to make all along. So much more was on the line than just emotions and fatigue. Katherine's future hung in the balance. She was giving every ounce of fight in her broken body and praying every prayer her broken lips could muster. I knew I needed to equip her to regain her life, even if it meant further delaying the homecoming for which my heart so longed. We would go home someday, just not yet.

As soon as I hung up the phone, my dad and I jumped in the car and drove directly to Casa Colina. Ironically, or perhaps as a God wink to us, Casa Colina looked more like the new apartment I had just moved into than like a hospital. Its grand entrance overflowed with bougainvillea, and the main road was lined with glorious palm trees. Its buildings and rooftops were colored a warm Mediterranean palette of taupes and terra-cottas. These first moments on the property softened the blow of knowing that a move here would be a move away from the Los Angeles community that had bolstered us for the past three and a half months, as well as a move into yet another hospital setting.

We sat with a bubbly admissions counselor who detailed the ins and outs of a potential stay. "Casa Colina's Transitional

Living Center is one of the best long-term neurological care facilities in the country," she recounted proudly. "Our Transitional Living Center helps survivors of all kinds of brain and spinal cord injuries transition into their new lives."

It was a comforting thought that Katherine might be prepared to come back home someday soon, but at the same time, a sense of loss lingered as I considered our options. "So the goal is not to help her recover but rather to help her learn how to live with her new limitations?" I choked out, feeling the stinging of new tears in the corner of my eyes.

"Well, it's both," she said sympathetically. "At this point in Katherine's recovery, no one knows what her long-term outcomes will be, but we want to help equip her to safely return to her new life, feeling confident in engaging you and her son, no matter what her recovery looks like."

This sounded reasonable enough, though it still felt like a defeat. *Can't they try harder to keep working with her therapy? She's so willing. She just needs more time*, I thought in exasperation.

"Jay, you should know we have a special housing program that would enable you and your son to live in a rental house next door to us, since Katherine would be living as an inpatient in the facility." This piece of the puzzle seemed like a godsend. I had no idea how we would commute nearly an hour from the new apartment in Los Angeles every day. I concluded that we would have to let go of the dream of living there as a family for a time until we could fully embrace this new opportunity.

"You should also know that our average stay at the Transitional Living Center, based on insurance approvals, is only sixty days."

As the previous months had demonstrated, I supposed we could do anything for a few months. The admissions coordinator toured us around the campus, passing pleasant garden alcoves and fountains sparkling in the bright midday sun.

Patients suffering from quadriplegia or neurological disorders, even loss of limbs, were the norm. Family members tended to their sick loved ones in this idyllic setting, the beauty of which did little to hide the fact that all was not well. These bittersweet vignettes of caregivers and patients both broke my heart in their vulnerability and yet made me feel like I had found a place where Katherine and James and I might belong in this next phase of our odyssey.

As we looked around the cafeteria, where Katherine would still, sadly, not be able to eat, my eyes caught a glimpse of a large Casa Colina banner above the exit. Upon reading the words a sizable lump formed in my throat: "The Miracle Continues." Suddenly this conflicted decision became very clear.

The tears came, and with them a deep assuredness that I had not felt before. Nearly four months ago, God had inexplicably given Katherine the miracle of survival. The ensuing months of slow-motion progress made it all too easy to overlook the miraculous nature of her recovery. How quickly we forget the miracles of our past as we step into an uncertain future, fearing we've used up our allotment of God's provision and we're all out of miracles. Katherine and I needed to be reminded of the miracles we had been given so we might remember the miracles to come, and we needed to find a place where the miracles could continue. It seemed we had found it at Casa Colina, though we had no idea what we would have to endure in order to see those miracles come to fruition.

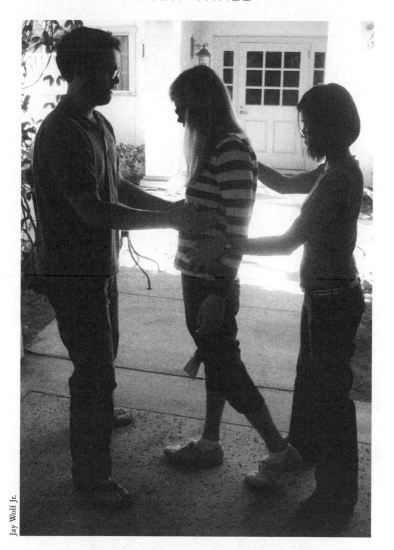

PART THREE

Jay Wolf Jr.

THE MIRACLE
CONTINUES

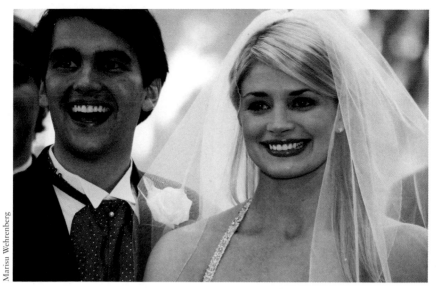

Marisu Wehrenberg

Wedding day (November 6, 2004)

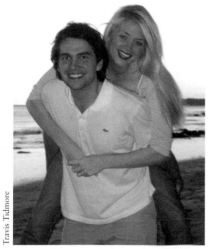

Travis Tidmore

Newlyweds in Malibu (August 2005)

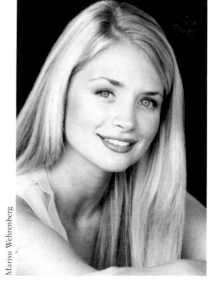

Marisu Wehrenberg

Katherine modeling (2005)

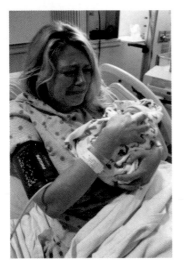

James's birth
(October 16, 2007)

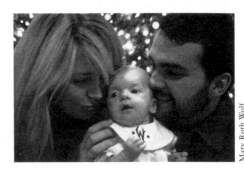

Mary Ruth Wolf

Christmas card with James
(December 2007)

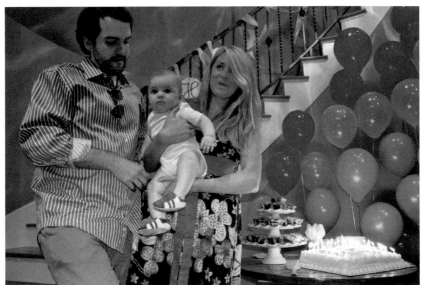

Ryan Daniel Dobson

Joint birthday party, three weeks before stroke (April 2008)

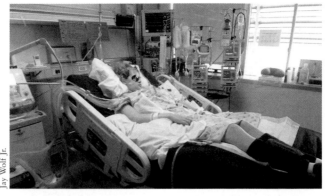

Katherine in UCLA's Intensive Care Unit (April 2008)

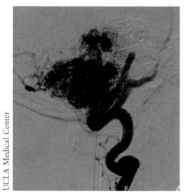

Presurgery, Katherine's
Arteriovenus Malformation
(AVM) (April 21, 2008)

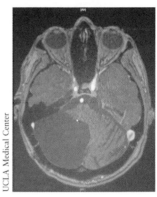

Postsurgery, partial removal
of Katherine's cerebellum
(April 22, 2008)

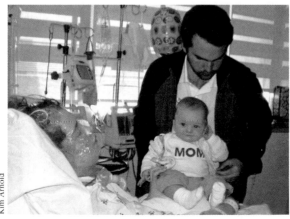

Katherine's first Mother's Day (May 2008)

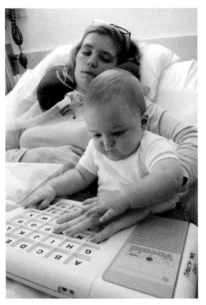

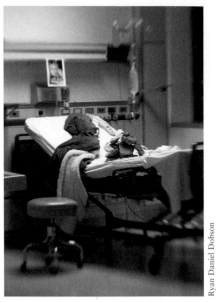

Ryan Daniel Dobson

UCLA's acute rehab unit with James
and letter board (July 2008)

Ebenezer stones in Katherine's
ICU bed (July 2008)

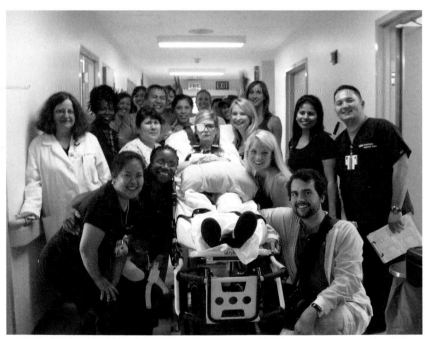

Good-bye to the UCLA Medical Center (August 2008)

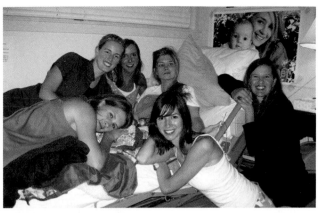

Small group friends visiting Casa Colina (September 2008)

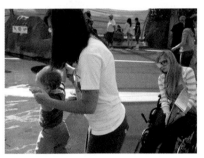

Casa Colina field trip with Sarah
and James (October 2008)

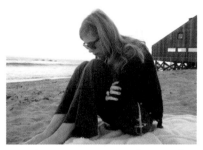

Fourth anniversary—Katherine's first
return to Malibu (November 2008)

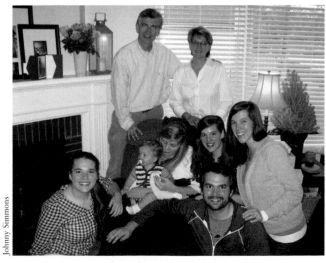

Johnny Simmons

"Epiphany of hope" moment (Thanksgiving 2008)

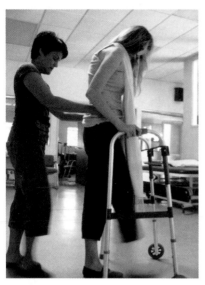

Casa Colina physical therapy
(January 2009)

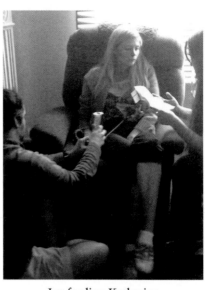

Jay feeding Katherine
through the g-tube (February 2009)

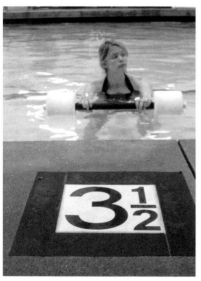

Casa Colina pool therapy
(Spring 2009)

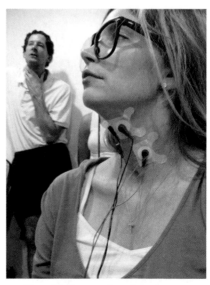

Casa Colina swallowing therapy
(Spring 2009)

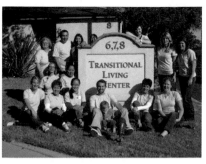

Good-bye to Casa Colina
(November 2009)

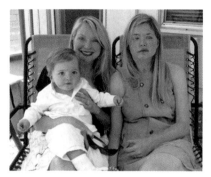

Mother's Day,
after first facial surgery (May 2009)

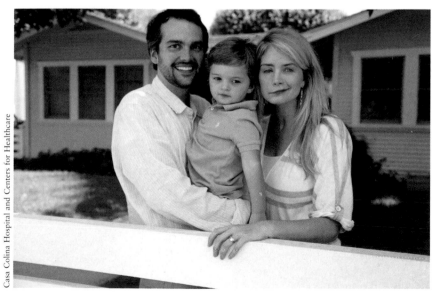

Casa Colina Hospital and Centers for Healthcare

At home in Culver City (Spring 2010)

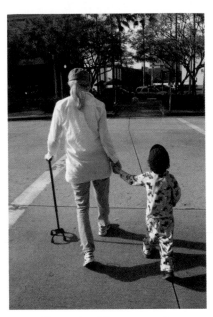

Becoming Mommy again
(November 2011)

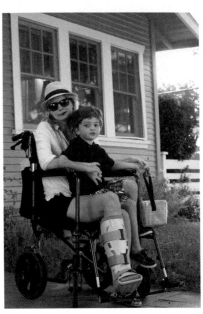

James's first day of kindergarten—
Katherine with broken leg
(August 2012)

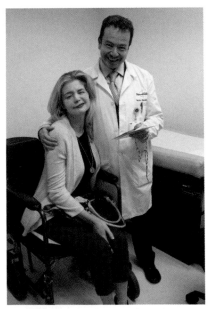

Dr. Gonzalez appointment after
aneurysm surgery (December 2013)

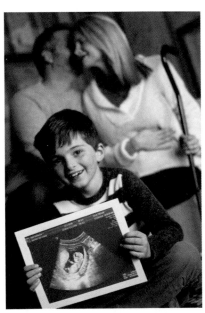

Pregnancy announcement
(January 2015)

Alex Wolf

Katherine

The decision had been made. It was time to move me to an inpatient facility for intensive brain rehabilitation.

The night before leaving the UCLA Medical Center, our small group gathered in my hospital room for a time of prayer and reflection on the past three and a half months. It had been an intense time of bonding and sacrifice, as these friends had led the charge for the greater community to rally around us. They knew their roles would change as we moved away from Los Angeles, and we all strangely mourned the end of the unique experience we had shared, though it had been one of the most difficult any of us had ever known.

Knowing that even the most life-changing experiences fade over time, Jay wanted to memorialize our stint at UCLA. Interestingly, the acute rehab ward was the only part of the hospital that had not moved across the street to a brand-new state-of-the-art medical facility. My original ICU room and the entire rest of the hospital, which had been abuzz with doctors and patients just a few weeks before, was now empty, so Jay and our friend Ryan ventured up to the eerily quiet seventh floor and set up a poignant re-creation of my ICU room. They gathered literal bricks from that old building's crumbling exterior as "Ebenezers"—stones of remembrance—as the Israelites had done to remind them of God's provision. Jay and Ryan stacked the bricks on the actual ICU bed on which I had lain for forty days and forty nights and photographed it.

We are all forgetful people—forgetful of our purpose, forgetful of who God is and what He has done. We need symbols of remembrance to be embodied in people and objects and visuals so we don't forget what certain experiences in our lives meant to us. That photograph would be one such reminder for Jay and me as we entered a new and unknown season, one in which we might easily succumb to fears and doubts. God had not left us then, and so we could trust He wasn't going to leave us in the future.

The next morning, I was transferred from my hospital bed to a stretcher to be transported to Casa Colina by ambulance. I wished I could have transitioned to this new stage of freedom in a more unrestrained fashion. I had pictured getting into my car, maybe like after my wedding reception, waving to the crowd as I went on to something new. But the reality was that I was too sick to even safely ride in a car. Once again, I would be taken on a stretcher via ambulance to somewhere unknown, to my new home.

As I was wheeled into the hallway, the flashing of cameras and loud applause caught me off guard. More than thirty friends and family members, nurses, technicians, therapists, and even several of my doctors had gathered to say good-bye. They would miss me. They would miss my constant stream of sweet visiting friends and family. But above all, they would miss Jay Wolf. They would miss watching the unfolding and epic love story of a young man's deep devotion to his bride. I'm sure they had seen far too much of the opposite, tragically. But Jay had demonstrated dedication and deep devotion to his crippled wife and crippled life. He was their daily, living word picture of what a true man looks like in a world full of scared, compassion-challenged little boys.

The people who worked on that floor would also miss Jay's kindness. Being treated with genuine care was not the norm for those folks. Most patients were so focused on their own pain and suffering that it was impossible for them to even consider loving and caring for their doctors or nurses or janitors or therapists. Jay took a genuine interest in these strangers and cared about making them feel special every day. On the morning of my departure, in a typical Jay Wolf display of love, he brought them Sprinkles cupcakes. Ever the celebration wizard, he assembled a three-tiered gorgeous display (he showed me pictures) in the break room, where the staff could indulge in a rainbow of flavors whenever they wanted. I recommended they try the dark chocolate—my favorite—in my honor.

As we were taken outside to meet the ambulance, the driver strapped me to the stretcher by my arms, feet, and middle. As I bid my final good-byes, I couldn't even wipe away the tears because my hands were tethered. By that point, helplessness was a feeling I had come to know all too well. As I was loaded into the ambulance, I saw the faces of my mom, sisters, and many sweet friends. As they waved, I tried to wave back, to smile and be brave, but the lump in my throat kept growing. On the inside, I was so very sad. All I wanted was to stay here and never leave, except to go back to my old life in Los Angeles, back to a life where there had never been a stroke or a surgery or a hospital.

Wait! Stop all this! I wanted to scream. *I don't want to go! Please don't make me go.* I wanted to get well, even if that meant moving to Antarctica, but I wanted the safety I had come to feel in acute rehab. *I know what to expect here. I'm scared to go somewhere new!*

But I had to go. They all knew it; I knew it too.

To my great relief, Jay was allowed to ride with me in the ambulance. Although we didn't speak very much through that weird and somber trip, we were both mentally preparing ourselves for what the coming hours would bring. And as we would almost immediately find out, the preparation would be desperately needed.

Joy

The summer night fell on Casa Colina with a soft dampness, like a warm towel not quite finished drying. The sounds of life settling down for sleep were certainly different than the ones you might hear in LA's city limits. Crickets sang and cicadas buzzed as I walked the hundred yards from our new rental home to the Transitional Living Center, "the TLC," where Katherine would do therapy during the day and stay the night from now on.

It had been a big day leaving UCLA and getting settled at Casa Colina, the third new microworld we had entered since the stroke. The folks who ran things seemed very professional and nice enough. I could only imagine their stress in working day in and day out with patients who were all living some variation of the worst nightmare of their lives. Everyone deemed suitable for this program had suffered some sort of neurological trauma, and while their deficits varied greatly, one common thread tied them together: They all stood on the precipice of despair, and this place was their last chance for hope.

Katherine would begin a whole new intensive level of therapy the next day, about which we were enthusiastic but nervous, but I had not anticipated a change that would be the hardest of all, for me at least. I would no longer be able to spend the night in Katherine's room. In the ICU, she had her own nurse 24/7, waiting and watching. In acute rehab, we had cobbled together that same 24/7 schedule with friends and family, which included someone spending the night in her room every night. This was mostly done so Katherine would know she was not alone. Now there would be no night watch, no one she could call for help if she needed something right away, no one to comfort her if she awoke from the nightmares that constantly plagued her.

I felt like a parent sending my baby off to camp for the first time—stomach-churning anticipation of new growth mixed with the sickening reality that she was effectively on her own now. The one comfort was that Katherine had been reunited with her cell phone. Despite her severe double vision and lack of her once-dominant right hand, she had relearned how to use her phone with her left hand for emergency purposes. It was her connection to the world. It would help communicate for her better than she could for herself, but it was still a poor substitute for a human companion.

I waved as I walked past the nurses' station and down the short hall that led to her new room. One of the main reasons I could not stay the night was that Katherine would now have a roommate. Charlotte was in her sixties, a petite, feisty-looking woman with short, cropped hair and glasses. At first glance, she could have been a teacher or someone's grandmother, but upon further observation, she fit neither of those descriptions. She walked around well enough, though slowly, limping due to the paralysis emanating from her left leg to the left arm that hung by her side. Her right hand was constantly roving her body, manically fishing in her pockets, down her pants, or on top of her head, as she muttered sternly to herself. She had suffered a stroke in the prefrontal region of her brain, as many at the TLC had; thus her cognition, memory, and emotions were in a state of flux. This was the only version of Charlotte we had known, but it was clearly not the one who had existed before her stroke. Needless to say, she was not exactly the bunkmate one would choose for their little camper.

That night, Katherine had been prepared for bed by the nursing assistants while Charlotte lingered in the large communal living area where residents could watch TV or just sit in their wheelchairs until it was time for bed. When I arrived at the room, Katherine was already tucked in, the foot of her bed covered by the handmade blanket from her ICU nurse's mom. We had wasted no time trying to make the place feel like home, tacking up dozens of photos and large signed cards and posters to cheer her up and make her feel a little more at home.

We held hands and sat in silence, until she began asking rapid-fire questions about the new rental house we were living in and in which she would have much rather been staying the night. Charlotte entered the room suddenly and plopped down on her bed, annoyed that I was there—but even more, that Katherine was there.

Earlier in the day, when we had first met Charlotte, Katherine eagerly introduced herself, almost childlike in her new, gravelly but once-again singsongy voice.

"Hi, how are ya?" she chipperly offered to her new room-mate and potential new best friend. Perhaps Charlotte would be a resource for some sage wisdom—or at least a safe person with whom Katherine could commiserate about their shared plight.

"What did you say?" Charlotte snapped back. "I can't understand you."

Bruised but undeterred, Katherine continued to engage her, asking questions about this new place and her background. Charlotte was not only uninterested in Katherine and her line of questions, but the whole situation seemed to irrationally agitate her in a way that terrified me. *What might she do? Could she hurt Katherine?* Katherine was still so impaired that she could barely hold her own head up, much less get into a wheelchair on her own.

"I want a divider in this room," Charlotte screamed out. "I don't want to see you!"

Katherine gasped audibly and began to choke back tears. It was the time she most needed a friend, but it was clear she would not find one in her new roommate.

I quickly wheeled her out of the room and asked the head

nurse to get a divider, per Charlotte's request—and now also per ours.

That experience in this new place was not the most comforting for Katherine to fall asleep thinking about on her first night, and that made me sad. Katherine and I held hands for a moment more. "It's going to be okay," I assured her.

"I'm not sure it is," Katherine said, her voice breaking as tears began to fall down her cheeks. "I don't want you to go."

"I don't want to go either," I stammered.

A nursing assistant appeared in the doorway. "Mr. Wolf, visiting hours are over now."

I slowly rose from Katherine's bedside, stooping over her for a good-night kiss. Katherine began to sob harder. I lingered, not wanting to leave.

"Mr. Wolf, we'll take good care of her."

I bent down again and whispered to Katherine, "Don't cry. Don't worry. I'll be back soon." She nodded silently, her tears subsiding a bit. The nursing assistant turned off the light as I left.

My tears came on hard as I walked quickly out the front door and into the night air. *O God, O God, what have I done? I thought this was the place You had for her? What have I done?*

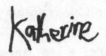

I woke up while it was still dark outside. There was a dim light on in the hallway of this strange new place, and I could see only a small amount in the large and sterile-looking room.

Where am I? Who is snoring over there? It doesn't sound like Jay. Why are we in separate beds?

Wait . . . this isn't my hospital bed. This is a regular

twin-sized bed, though. Am I back at summer camp? Am I back home? What's going on? I'm so confused.

Then it all came back to me. *This isn't a bad dream. I'm really in this terrifying place, and scary Charlotte is actually my roommate. I've got to get out of here.* Charlotte's bizarre, manic reaching into her pants and pockets and frantically searching her body for something had me flipping out that she would try to do the same to me in my sleep. I lay very still in the darkness as the morning slowly lit up our room. Charlotte kept snoring. I was not about to wake her up.

All of a sudden, the lights came on, and a perky thirty-something female was standing over me. "Good morning! We shower every patient every morning here, so I will be helping you take off all your clothes, and then I'll wheel you into the line in the hallway for a shower. Don't worry. I'll put a towel over you before we leave the room."

Um, I'm sorry, what? She can't be serious about this. There is no way I'm doing any of that. Does my family know about this? Has anyone okayed this with Jay?

Though I had been physically cared for by others for months, I had been sponge bathed only in the privacy of my own room. I didn't know these new people, and I didn't know where they would be taking me or why I needed to be nude first. Would there be nude men in the hallway too? The aide began unbuttoning my pajama top, exposing my breasts while I just sat there.

I suddenly had an idea of how to get myself out of this craziness. With my voice shaking, I choked out, "Wait! I don't need to shower every day. I don't wash my hair every morning at home anyway. I can't walk right now and don't sweat much these days, so I can just wait and take a shower tomorrow. I'll be fine without doing it today. Thank you, though. I really appreciate it."

"I'm sorry," she said, the quizzical look on her face communicating that she didn't understand what I thought was a very clear declaration. "It is policy here that every patient takes a morning shower every day. We will need to take off your pants and underwear and transfer you to your wheelchair now."

All I could do was watch in horror as she pulled off my pajama pants and underwear. I started crying as she transferred me to my wheelchair. She lovingly patted my back as she draped a large towel around me, fully covering my nude body.

After waiting my turn in line, I was wheeled into the shower and allowed to lather my own hair for the first time in almost four months. It was dignifying yet jarring, as I could only wash and lather with my left hand, and it took twice as long as normal. But those uninterrupted moments in the shower were my first real moments of privacy since the stroke. *O God, can this be real?* I knew I wasn't the only one virtually in shock at where I found myself that morning. I'm sure everyone in that hallway—wrapped in towels, many of whom were crying too—were in pain and disbelief, just like I was. None of us asked to be there, and none of us could change the fact that we were there.

As hot water and tears streamed down my face, I resolved to work my hardest in therapy so I could get out of there as soon as possible. I also decided to not let my circumstances make me bitter and hopeless. I wanted to be able to encourage and inspire this new community, just like I did at the UCLA Medical Center.

By the time Jay arrived, two aides playing beauty parlor had done my hair and finished my makeup, and I was ready to attend my first therapy session at Casa Colina. I had no idea what to expect. I was anxious to get my schedule and find out how my new therapies would work in this place. I had had only private therapy at UCLA; here I would be in group sessions.

This first hour was called "Disability Adjustment." As Jay wheeled me into a large room with a massive table for the patients, he carefully navigated around the fifteen or so other wheelchairs in the room. There were about forty people total,

and many did not look very impaired. There were several inter-
preters for non-English speaking patients, and the racket made
concentrating on the teacher's words very difficult.

"Let's start by writing your name. Please write first and
last. Then write the date with the year. Then write the name of
our current president and what state we are in right now." After
easily answering the questions, I waited for several minutes.
*Why was this taking so long? These were such basic questions
that anyone could answer.*

"Okay, next I would like you to go around and answer
out loud, 'What is trauma?' You have all had a trauma to
your brain. Let's go around and say what our trauma was for
everyone to hear."

I felt like I had been transplanted into a very sad prison of
sorts that was full of people in the worst spots of their lives. I
was surprised by the large number of traumatic brain injuries
due to accidents of all kinds. There were race car accidents, car
wrecks, motorcycle wrecks, horseback-riding accidents, falling-
off-a-ladder accidents, several shootings. Still other patients had
diseases or trauma that hadn't resulted from sudden injuries.
There were folks with ALS, cerebral palsy, and multiple scle-
rosis; amputees; and severely diabetic patients who were blind
and unable to walk. One woman had suffered a stroke from an
AVM rupture, as I had, but hers had affected a slightly different
part of the brain, and the damage was all cognitive. While her
body was fine and she looked "normal," she could no longer
read or write. She would hold up three fingers and say "apple."
I could sense that she knew something was very wrong and was
desperate to relearn numbers and letters. I knew how easily that
could have been me.

By far the most striking patient to me was Danny. He foamed
at the mouth and was more like a six-foot-three two-year-old
than a man. He had been hit in the head with a baseball bat

by intruders while trying to protect his mother, and now he couldn't even recognize her. He had two techs with him at all times for the safety of the other patients. Though normally quite calm and childlike, he was prone to occasional violent outbursts, his long arms flailing as he screamed in frustration, having no words to explain his pain. It was horrifying to see other human beings who no longer understood how to be human.

There were so many variations of terrible, life-altering anguish here. Suffering was all around me. So why did I feel so alone in my pain? Perhaps the feelings of isolation stemmed from the fact that I was one of the youngest patients at Casa Colina, and I'd found out the previous day that I was the only patient who couldn't swallow. I knew lunch was coming, and all these wheelchair-clad people could load up a tray with good ole cafeteria eats while I could only sit by and watch.

My mother, my sister, my aunt, and Jay brought James to visit for my first lunch hour as a blessed distraction. My sweet family tried so hard to make this better for me. They knew this new place, especially at mealtime, had to be the stuff of nightmares for me. Seeing my big-eyed cutie did make the day somewhat better, but nothing could really help make my sad reality more tolerable.

After a foodless "lunch" and other therapies, I ended my day with a group class called "Cognitive Reasoning." I left in tears, feeling crazy.

I don't belong. I'm the same as before in my head. Does no one get that? My brain was hurt, but I don't think my cognitive mind is messed up. Or is it, and I'm just in denial? Were all my answers just good guesses? I think I'm the same . . . I don't know for sure, though. Am I crazy? No . . . but what if no one believes me?

As Jay wheeled me up to my room, I felt defeated. My shower pep talk from that morning seemed like a joke. My room looked so sad—like a prison—and the smell of antiseptic was disgusting. Just then, I had one of the more depressing realizations of my entire ordeal: *All of these characters are my new peer group.*

I thought about my life before this hell. I was with my former peer group—the law school new mommies playing on the beach with our babies, or the sweet gals from church laughing and gabbing a mile a minute. I tried not to cry too loudly as I braced myself for another night with Charlotte.

Jay

We plunged into a new routine and a new period of darkness. In contrast to our previous therapy experiences, Casa Colina's niche was for patients who needed longer-term care, so these patients were worse off than those in acute rehab. It was clear that the light at the end of the tunnel was growing dimmer for them. Broken brains and broken hopes filled the place with a palpable heaviness and an aroma of sorrow.

Once during that first week, we were late to an early therapy session, so I pushed Katherine up an incline at a quick pace, nodding a silent greeting to a large, middle-aged man in a wheelchair, with an amputated leg, whom I thought was just waiting at the bottom. Apparently, I had cut him off.

"F*?# you!" he screamed. "You a**hole! Who do you think you are?!"

Katherine gasped, embarrassed and horrified. I was so flabbergasted that I could barely stutter out an "I'm sorry" before moving ahead quickly as he continued to mutter expletives in the background. I felt bad for slighting him, but more than that, I felt angry. His words slapped Katherine's broken spirit in a way I knew I had to protect her from.

I started to see what happens when a group of people in

horrific physical and emotional pain are placed together in a small space and are pushed to recover the things they have lost, while you grieve with them for the things they will never recover. A compounded, collective sense of loss lingers like a heavy fog over everything. We were not recovering in a vacuum, alone; this recovery would be entangled, communal. But as unfair as that seemed, perhaps if the pain is shared, some hope may be also.

The physical therapy gym where all the patients commingled on padded benches with balls and harnesses was similar to UCLA's surgical waiting room in that there was nowhere to hide one's raw struggles, nor was there a way to avoid encountering the pain of others. Grown quadriplegic men wept in despair as their aged parent caregivers joined in silent lamentation. Cries of physical pain often pierced the air as patients tried once-normal movements they could no longer perform. Yet also like the waiting room, we had an opportunity to share in the pain of others and to offer the comfort we had received. Often the simplest course of action was to confront this communal suffering head-on, which Katherine did with determination and grace. She would place her hand on the shoulder of a fellow patient and speak truth into their tears. Though her words were garbled, her love was clear.

Blessedly, in the midst of this dark covering of grief were bright pinpricks of light from the tireless efforts of the therapists, techs, and doctors. Their work was miraculous, not necessarily in the outcomes as much as in the dailyness of their resolve to walk with their patients through the journey of suffering. It was clear that emotional healing was perhaps the deepest need for everyone there. And maybe if the healing of the heart began, it could pave the way for hope for the future, enough hope to engage the unbearable grind necessary for physical healing.

The staff became fast friends with our family, as Katherine connected with them in a way few of their patients could. Unlike many of the cognitively injured patients, she was kind and interested in the lives of her therapists, and unlike many of her new peers struggling in despair, she was hopeful and motivated to give each session of therapy her absolute best effort.

I accompanied Katherine to almost all of her sessions—swallowing, speech, physical, and occupational therapies—though after a few weeks, I felt comfortable enough with her new team to allow them to do their work without me at times. I began to spend more time with James, who was still being cared for by my sister Sarah. He was rapidly approaching his first birthday and was getting close to taking his first step, while it seemed his mommy was still a long way from taking hers.

As Katherine resolved to live fearlessly in her new peer group, it made my heart proud while making it break as well. The same vibrancy still exuded through the shell of her body, but it was painful to watch a woman who had never met a stranger and had always been comfortable in her own skin become increasingly self-conscious, even shamed, by the constraints of her new body, voice, and appearance. I had a deep desire to help Katherine regain some of the dignity lost by virtue of being disabled and living in a hospital. Her awareness of her new self and her interaction with others were much greater than at UCLA, so we felt the need to somehow empower her as she engaged the unglamorous and mundane world of therapy.

In true Southern-belle style, her mom had equipped us with a new and improved bevy of beauty tools, makeup, and hair curlers, which she helped Katherine use when she was in town, or the techs helped with when they had time to play beauty salon in the early mornings while getting Katherine ready for the day. Yet this task more often than not fell on me. Though I have three sisters, I had no hands-on experience with these specifically female practices. My first attempts at doing Katherine's hair and makeup were so pitiful that I nearly decided to never undertake them again. If the purpose was to dignify Katherine, then giving her the appearance of an electrocuted clown was not going to be very helpful! After much practice, however, I began to learn my way around a hair straightener and an eyebrow pencil. My work was not exactly of the caliber for which one might pay money or be a repeat customer, but it seemed my only repeat customer had little choice in the matter.

I also realized that Katherine had bought literally no clothes since we had gotten married almost four years before. She had received hand-me-ups from her younger sisters, who were much more into shopping than she was. At this juncture, she had lost nearly thirty pounds since her stroke, so most of her clothes hung loosely on her new frame. I went to the nearby mall, getting annoyed stares from women wandering the same sale section aisles on which I had encroached. Having never purchased female clothing without the wearer present, I eye-balled things I thought might fit Katherine, garments in which she might feel both comfortable and pretty, and excitedly took my purchases back for her approval. My efforts at fashion and makeup helped more than they hurt, and at the very least, they showed Katherine that every part of her mattered, even these non-life-and-death parts, because every part of her was loved.

As I drove home, I popped a CD in without looking at it. With the first strains, I recognized it. Each year, we made a music playlist for the joint birthday party we threw each other, and we burned CD copies as our signature party favor. This playlist was from the most recent party, thrown just three weeks before the stroke, and it had a particular poignancy because it was inspired by James's fairly recent arrival. These songs about new life and family had been our soundtrack in the weeks before everything changed. As the songs played in familiar succession, I was transported in time in the way only music can do. In that juxtaposed moment of a life that had been and a new, very different life that was, my heart broke at the loss so profoundly that I began to cry and yell so uncontrollably that I feared I would have to pull off the interstate.

It's easy to look the other way when confronted with grief or to busy oneself so as to not sit with grief long. Yet somehow in the solitude of my car, music began to remove the stitches I had used to quickly sew up my heart and shore up my grief. To my surprise, in this unraveling I didn't find myself undone, but rather, like glimpsing a wound under an old bandage, I could not deny that I was healing. I was learning more about love than three years of marriage might normally teach. I was learning that vulnerability and grief were love's inevitable companions.

I realized why Katherine had always promoted the necessity of a good "hormonal scream cry" in the bathtub every now and then. These groans articulated far more than my prayers could have, and the sense of peace I felt afterward transcended most peace I had ever experienced. In the past few months, I had shed more tears than in the combined total of all my previous years, and yet I knew they were not wasted. I knew God saw them and even counted them. He heard my cries, and He was going to rescue us. To know you will be saved, even if you don't dare envision how, is to have the wick of hope kindled.

Perhaps my crying sessions were more evident than I thought, because the Casa Colina social worker encouraged me to check out a community fitness center, which had pools and workout classes and child care, and I began to force myself to go there. I felt guilty most times and kept an anxious eye on the clock, not wanting to be late for Katherine's next therapy session or break, but it felt undeniably good every time I channeled my stress into physical exertion. I wished stress naturally led me to loss of appetite and the need to take a marathon jog, but it was much more natural for me to seek respite and distraction in TV, busyness, food, or alcohol. Though I had always managed stress well, at least externally, it was clear that the level of stress in my life now needed somewhere else to go. I began to realize that this is the challenging balance for the caregiver: How can you "put the oxygen mask on yourself first," so to speak, when it feels like the least natural thing to do? It makes sense in theory, but in practice, it's profoundly difficult because it costs both the caregiver and the patient. Yet practicing some routines of self-care would be essential to walking with Katherine for the long haul.

We went to therapy all morning and afternoon and then hung out in her room until bedtime. It was a grueling schedule, but at least I got to go home at the end, unlike Katherine, who almost never left the building. Given our unique situation of living next to the hospital, I proposed a new afternoon activity to our friends who ran the TLC. I would take Katherine directly from her last therapy session back to our rental home and then return her to her room by evening so she could spend the night at the facility. They allowed this simple bending of the rules, and it bent our hope back into alignment too. It was a small shift in schedule and location, but the ripple effects would change everything. Instead of spending her free time consigned to the communal TV or her room and unfriendly roommate, she would now be able to pretend she was living a normal life with me and James, if only for a few short hours. These precious afternoons would be the vital fuel for the battle that lay ahead for her.

The first time I wheeled Katherine off campus the short distance to our house, I was giddy. It had become more and more difficult to live with spontaneity and joy when life's fragility had been made so painfully obvious to us. And yet we needed to begin safely risking again and, in so doing, be reminded of the profound gift Katherine had received in this second chance to live. I proudly wheeled her up the ramp to the very accessible house. It was fairly small and kind of shabby around the edges, but it represented a core truth to which we would cling: Don't wait to celebrate the life you have been given, even if it looks different from the one you thought you would have. This place would be our new home, even though we felt like we were anywhere but home.

I had brought quite a few reminders of our Pepperdine apartment to this house, including a painting Katherine had given me, a favorite lamp, and the framed wedding pictures that had always lived on our bedside tables, including the image that both haunted me and sowed hope in me—the picture of Katherine joyfully running in her wedding dress. Katherine nearly jumped out of her wheelchair with delight, like a prisoner first stepping foot outside the walls. She claimed a prominent place on the living room couch, propped up to view the goings-on in the main room of the house. It was her first time to sit on a couch in four months. It was clear that this new experience left her feeling a bit self-conscious and uncomfortable, like a stranger in her old life, but those feelings began to noticeably evaporate as soon as she saw James and was able to engage him in this home setting rather than in the hospital. She quickly began to see that she was home and had a place to belong in this new life with us.

Katherine

After being at Casa Colina for only about a week, some of the women were (mostly) delighted to attend a "field trip" to the nail salon. This group of women was due for an outing both to engage "the real world" and to practice "daily life skills," such as paying for the services, following instructions, and interacting with people outside the hospital.

We boarded a short bus for our outing. I had a surreal moment of recognizing that this was "my" bus now. Loading seemed to take more than an hour because of all the wheelchairs and medical devices. My mom came with me, and I was delighted she was there. She could help communicate for me and was another fully able-bodied person. Other than Mom, I barely knew the other women and techs who joined us. Charlotte was there, and she did not speak to me the entire day. It was clear that this outing was highly stressful for her.

Once we finally left Casa Colina and turned onto the open road, I realized that this was the first time I had seen a road, trees, traffic signals, or much of anything else in more than five months. When I had been driven to Casa, I was on a stretcher and could not see outside. Now I was sitting upright and could see the world outside of brain injury, hospitals, and terrible suffering. I felt refreshed to see life happening outside the hospital walls.

However, I felt a deep sadness that I was no longer engaged with this world. I had memories of meeting other young mothers in the nail salon and plopping our babies beside us in their carriers while they napped peacefully. Now I was without my little sidekick, but with many new cohorts. My heart ached.

The nail services were clearly taxing and traumatic for most of the women. It was very difficult for the women performing these services as well. One patient saw spiders crawling up her arm while getting a manicure. Another patient thought the nail technicians were plotting to kill us and refused all services. Charlotte began taking off her pants in preparation for her pedicure. The whole scene was like a crazy circus, almost comical yet deeply disturbing.

The lowest point of the day came when my nail technician asked me five little words: "Were you born this way?"

I didn't understand what she could be referring to. Then I realized she meant my very shaky right hand, my wheelchair, and my paralyzed face.

"She had a massive stroke a few months ago," my mom quickly answered. This seemed to satisfy the technician as she tried to be delicate with my hands.

"You are doing great," the woman told me sympathetically (as everyone always told me). "You will keep getting better."

I certainly hope so, I thought as I looked around at our sad scene and my bizarre new reality. *Yes, I pray so.*

Jay

The greatest struggle for peace is always the internal one. Yet in the milieu of brain rehab, like any battle fought communally with fellow strugglers, the internal conflicts often cannot be contained within. Pain comes at everyone from all sides, and peace feels more and more remote.

Neil became a patient at Casa Colina, his trach scar still pink in the healing. He was our age but wore a permanent scowl under a hipster mustache. He had been under the influence of a number of illicit drugs when his car crashed and nearly killed him, leaving him with an injury to the frontal region of his brain. He was in physical pain from the crash, and while he was impaired, he was able to weakly hobble and sulk around the therapy gym. Often his pain manifested in a dark and unhinged violence, and he would unleash a barrage of profanity at any therapist who pushed him physically. Katherine was often in the same room with Neil during these outbursts.

One day, he let loose a particularly foul rant on his long-suffering therapist, accentuating his curses by spitting on her. Katherine had absolutely had enough and yelled, "Neil, stop it right now! You are disrespecting the person trying to help you!" Katherine thought such an admonition from a fellow patient might break through to Neil. Instead, his ire turned to her.

"You shut up, you b#@*h," he barked. "I can't even under-stand you. Your voice is always gonna be messed up, and so is your body!"

Katherine stood her ground with an authority that belied the deep wound caused by his words. "No, I am going to get better, Neil. And so are you."

I had never been more awestruck and proud to witness Katherine's true character shine in the face of such opposition.

She was winning her internal struggle for peace as Neil's internal resignation to war spewed out as rage. The conflict between them was real, yet the light would not be overcome.

Our negative interactions with Neil paled in comparison to our experiences with Tiffany, who arrived at Casa Colina just a few days after we did. She was our age but had a childlike quality about her, an arrested development resulting from a brain injury after a horse kicked her in the head when she was thirteen. She quickly cozied up to Katherine in their therapy session. Katherine saw a young-seeming, scared girl who needed a friend. Yet in the span of a few hours, Katherine experienced a bizarre and frightening reversal as Tiffany melted down after losing a group therapy card game. Katherine called me that night, terrified, as Tiffany, whose room was next to hers, began throwing her chair against the wall in a fit of rage. The situation was managed by the hospital staff, and Tiffany was assigned a 24/7 aide. But something changed that night.

The next time I wheeled Katherine past Tiffany in the hallway, Tiffany began to scream and cry uncontrollably, pointing a shaky finger at us, yelling profanity until her therapist wheeled her away. A few days later as I tucked Katherine in for the night, she tearfully recounted that Tiffany had whispered to her that I had raped Tiffany and she was now pregnant with my baby. While this story was disgustingly preposterous, it was a particularly low blow to Katherine, who was struggling with the realization that she greatly desired more children but may never be able to have them. I was flustered and furious, vowing to get to the bottom of this story the next day. As I was quickly walking out of the TLC, I passed Tiffany's room, averting my eyes from her cracked doorway. As I neared the end of the hall, Tiffany's shaky, brain-injured voice rang out with surprising clarity: "Good night, a**hole."

I discussed the situation with the TLC's psychiatrist in hopes of understanding why Tiffany might be focusing on

Katherine and me. She ascertained that some visual trigger, maybe Katherine's blonde hair or my beard, might be making a false neural connection in Tiffany's brain, reminding her of someone she used to know or someone she made up. There was no satisfying answer, and while we felt empathetic toward every patient suffering through the indignity of brain trauma, we began to sense a great darkness in our interactions with Tiffany. To be walking through a personal hell only to have someone else's thrust on you is nearly too much to bear. We walked on eggshells whenever Tiffany was around, avoiding eye contact, not engaging her at all. We began to resent the salt she was rubbing in our wounds, and we prayed the situation would change.

Early one morning, I received a call from Katherine, who excitedly recounted, "Tiffany's gone! Her parents came and got her late last night."

The relief was palpable around the TLC, as Tiffany's tumultuous, broken presence was notably absent. Yet as with every interaction in that place, there was a mixture of joy and sorrow because this stopped so far short of the kind of resolution that was most needed. We were all in need of rescue, even the ones holding us captive.

As fall came and the California permaclimate shifted to a subtly cooler version of itself, we felt something shifting inside too. Katherine had been making some wonderful improvements in her physical strength, and she continued to enjoy a healing respite in the daily afternoon visits to our house. Naturally, these visits began to lengthen, so much so that we found ourselves having to sneak back into the facility at night, like teenagers breaking curfew. Thankfully, a patient from across the hall left, so Katherine was cleared to move out of the room with Charlotte and into a private room once again. The techs smiled and turned a blind eye to our nightly covert operation because they loved Katherine and were rooting for her. They all knew the best medicine she could get was time with James and me, planting the seed of hope and home deep within her and giving her the strength to push through the monotonous, daily hell of therapy.

Since Katherine had made so much progress, we felt she could consider more reentry into the land of the living outside the hospital bubble. We had been out of church community for five months, the longest absence in our entire lives, and we felt it. Church had always been an indispensable part of who we were, a safe place for us. Katherine had been unable to return for medical reasons, but I had resisted returning because, for me, the communal experience of God, like the communal experience of therapy, brought with it a colliding, compounding effect for which I was not sure I was emotionally ready. I truly felt no anger toward God when I experienced Him alone, but I knew that reconnecting to the church would mean reengaging God in a different, deeper way—and there would be no turning back from the hard questions and the gift of His grace. Funny how we can sense the potential impact that the love of God will awaken within, and it scares us. It can be so painfully hard to receive that love because in the receiving we are confronted with our inability to gain it. Even as I was giving out my love to Katherine as a caregiver in a way she could not repay, I was challenged by the revelation that this is what God was doing for me. Could I receive His love, knowing I could never repay it?

My mom, who was staying with us at that time, researched a local church, Pomona First Baptist, which had an excellent kids' ministry that James could attend, and she began taking him for a few Sundays until we decided to join her. Katherine had been deemed well enough to leave the hospital campus for nearby destinations for short time periods, so I signed her out for the morning, and we headed to church. This church was large but earnest in its communication of the gospel and its desire to connect with the community. In many ways, it was quite different from other churches we had been a part of, yet the experience of encountering the same God we had always encountered before was comforting. We felt welcome, though we hardly felt at home yet. We sat in the back row, where Katherine's wheelchair could easily slip into an open space. We were warmly greeted, but we slipped out quickly after the service ended each week. Though we were seeing the great impact our story was making on a digital audience, we didn't yet have the words or courage to vulnerably share our deepest tragedy face-to-face with other humans. The wounds were too fresh to seek that type of exposure yet.

Emboldened by this reentry into the world and aware that we had more leeway than most inpatients at Casa Colina, we embarked on our biggest adventure yet. Our friends Andy and Anna were expecting the birth of their son at any moment, and Katherine was determined to show her support just as she would have before. A phone call or letter would not do. Katherine wanted to see Anna in person. Such a field trip surely wouldn't be approved by the rehab powers that be, so we implied that we would be hanging out at my house next door to the hospital for the evening.

As I loaded Katherine into the car, I began to second-guess our impulsive decision. She insisted, unwaveringly, and threatened to hitchhike there if I refused to take her to the hospital where Anna was to give birth, so I complied. I drove the fifty miles back to LA as one would drive home from the hospital with a newborn, my hands gripping the steering wheel tightly, my awareness heightened to every car around us. I was nervous but felt this calculated risk was worth it, necessary even. Katherine had gained a greater realization of all she had lost in recent weeks, and this sense of loss was heightened as it became clear that life in our LA community was naturally moving on without us. Milestones were celebrated, and babies were being born—and we were not there. Katherine longed to "do life together" again with our friends, and at that very moment, she wanted to be there for Anna in the way Anna had been there for her by caring for James in the weeks after the stroke. It was a small offering but an important one because Katherine was giving everything she had.

We surrounded Anna's bedside in the delivery room, soaking in the profound holiness of the moment. Our friends had long desired a baby, and we'd been praying for that for years. To confront this achingly beautiful cycle of new life and near death, severe loss and second chances, was to see the miracle of it all in a new way, and we cried tears of wonder and gratitude. We missed the baby's actual arrival, but we sped back to Casa Colina, far past curfew, in the afterglow of a night that was life-giving in every sense of the word.

A few days later, still encouraged by our successful trip into LA, we decided we would return to our home church, Bel Air Presbyterian, for a Sunday morning service. The next Sunday seemed apropos, as our beloved Young Marrieds group was having its fall kickoff. We didn't tell anyone of our plans, just in case the plans were to shift. We were excited but a little nervous to return. Could things ever be the same now that we were so different?

We woke up early, and I helped Katherine get ready, putting her makeup on her and doing her hair with special care. We made the hour-long trek and arrived a little late. I was still learning how to travel with the wheelchair and get Katherine in and out of the car, but our tardiness might actually make it easier than coming in at peak time when people would be streaming in around us. We entered the back door of the large room where the Young Marrieds met, my sister Sarah and James in tow, and I wheeled Katherine in just as our friends and mentors JT and Sydney were introducing the leadership team. In mid-sentence, they saw us and were so caught by surprise that they both burst into tears. The room erupted in a standing ovation and cheers. So much for inconspicuously slipping in the back!

We felt like Lazarus returning home after his resurrection, celebrating at an impromptu party all the more joyous for its heartfelt spontaneity. Friends surrounded and hugged us, weeping with delight to see the gospel embodied in flesh and blood in a way they had never encountered before—life when there should have been death. This community of Christ stood utterly amazed at what He had done, and in their amazement, our downtrodden gaze was lifted, as if by the hand of God, to His face. And we were amazed too.

Katherine

The ensuing weeks were arduous yet mundane, very difficult yet very boring at the same time. I kept getting approved by insurance to stay on at Casa Colina, while other patients came and left. This only highlighted what a bad-off case I was at that point.

My swallowing therapy seemed to get me nowhere. I would work five days a week for an hour each day on my swallow and wasn't able to gain a bit of progress. I would do special exercises inside and outside of class, and I was even getting electrical stimulation on my throat. None of it seemed to help.

Not eating was not getting any easier with time. I started to daydream about food every moment of the day. Thoughts of food would consume me while I did everything *but* eat. I would see a commercial for food on TV, and my mouth would salivate and I'd have epic cravings. I would purposefully spill some baby food on my wrist while feeding James and then lick my hand, savor the taste, and spit it back out. I was obsessed with swallowing again.

I harassed my speech therapist daily about my condition.

"When do you think I will swallow again?"

"Are there other people here who don't swallow?"

"Just how rare is it to not be able to swallow?"

"What is the average time people like me go without eating?"

"Are you sure I can't swallow? How can you be totally sure? Test results aren't always accurate."

She wisely did not engage any of these questions. She told me I was a unique case and that we would just have to keep working my swallowing muscles every day and hope for the best.

But there was a bright spot. After more than two and a half months of living as an inpatient at the Transitional Living Center, I was allowed to move into the house that my family was renting next door to the facility. It was a glorious change! Now I would get to enjoy James whenever I wasn't in therapy, and I also was safe in bed with Jay at night. It was a game changer in my ordeal, a turning point in my recovery.

After just five days of living at the house, we had a huge first birthday party for James. We had more than eighty-five people in the backyard of our little brain rehab house, mostly from our Los Angeles community more than an hour away, and I was deeply touched to see how well these friends still loved and supported us. Our party theme (we always had a theme) was "Life's a Zoo Because It Is." All the kids were dressed as zoo animals. James was the cutest little lion I had ever seen! We had a massive sheet cake, and I put my fingertip in the frosting and popped it into my mouth reflexively. The sugar melted on my tongue and slid down my throat. It wasn't exactly a swallow, but I didn't cough, so it must have gone down the right pipe!

It was so appropriate that my first taste of sweetness was on my son's first birthday . . . HEAVEN!

⚓

While in occupational therapy, I was encouraged to start writing cards again. They had a large stockpile of old cards, and most patients did not take advantage of the free stationery! Some women have a thing for shoes; I have always had a thing for monogrammed stationery. I had a whole closet at our old apartment dedicated to my stationery collection. I have loved writing cards or letters since I learned to write. As a child, I used to send my grandparents letters in the mail all the time, even though we lived in the same neighborhood.

I had received an insane amount of mail since my stroke. *I can begin writing people back!* I thought. *I will make note writing my purpose during this dark time. I have an outlet now. I can bless people with cards from my shaky hand.*

My first card was to Jay. It was a thank-you note for what he had done in the past six months. He could only tell it was a thank-you note because the word *thank* was the only legible word on the entire card! I could not coordinate my right hand's movements enough to write words that anyone (including myself) could decipher. Still, it conveyed a fraction of my gratitude to this man who never stopped showing me what real love looked like.

He had been affected by everything I was going through as deeply as if he had had the brain injury himself. He grieved as deeply as I did and let me mourn. When I cried myself to sleep at night, he just put his arms around me and whispered that everything was going to be all right.

In addition to going to every therapy session, he did so many things any man should never have to do, much less one at our age. He flossed my teeth, put on my lipstick, fed me all my "food" and medications through a tube, lifted me on and off every machine at the gym, brushed and blow-dried my hair, picked out my outfits every morning and dressed me before therapy, put on my deodorant, took me to the bathroom *every single time* I had to go, and even shaved my armpits. Now that's love! Even if we were in the middle of an argument (yes, we still argued), he had to put ointment on my scars or lube in my bad eye. The physicality of our interaction was an ongoing lesson of sacrificial love.

Jay also had to become "Mr. Mom," and he embraced the role. Even with his sister and both our moms working like dogs to care for our little one, Jay spent quality time with James every day. Even after being with me in therapy all day, he played with our little guy afterward. For James's first birthday party, he addressed the invitations and wrote thank-you cards for all the gifts. He took over the care of our little house, lovingly making it a place of comfort and beauty. He even began teaching himself to cook, even though I couldn't eat yet. He said he was perfecting his skills for the day when I would finally be able to join him and James at the dinner table.

Jay loved me without asking for anything in return. I felt so uncomfortable, so unlovely, in my new skin, yet he made me feel beautiful and desirable. It was a process to relearn how to be vulnerable and intimate, since we were in every way very different people than we were before the stroke. Jay helped me remember who I was in the deepest parts of me. He showed me that true love means he did not want anything from me; he just loved me freely, just as I was. His true love was my hand to hold through my darkest valley.

Jay was a great man before (I did marry him, after all), but now I'd seen much more than met the eye in that Alabama fraternity boy. It was a blessing to me that the world was getting to see what I had seen all along.

Jay

Nearly seven months into our ordeal, we celebrated our fourth wedding anniversary. As I walked Katherine back from an early morning trip to the bathroom, I rigged our wedding DVD to start playing at the bridal procession. After a few seconds, the strains of "Trumpet Voluntary" ignited memories in Katherine's mind, sending a sweet, crooked smile across her face. I knew that Katherine's "procession" this morning, though in a bathrobe with her eye patched, was far more beautiful than her walk down the aisle on our wedding day.

We continued to slowly make our way back to the bed in the familiar, swaying dance/walk that we found ourselves in every day now—my hands on her hips, her hands on my shoulders, my feet spread wide to balance us both. Memories of how we danced to the band for hours at our reception came racing back. Even if we wouldn't be dancing that way for a while, I got to lead my wife in a new kind of dance all the time.

We lay in bed watching the wedding DVD before getting ready for our day of therapy. The two people on the screen were so young, so innocent. The bride, though now unable to walk down any aisle or clearly speak her wedding vows or eat her beloved wedding cake, was somehow, impossibly more radiant than she was then. Now she glowed with the light of life restored. We had been battered, but we were not broken. We had experienced things that two twentysomethings should never have to experience, but we had also been filled to overflowing with the immeasurable blessings of our Lord.

As we listened to my dad's words preceding the vows at our wedding ceremony, we could not help but transport ourselves back to the moments on that altar. My dad had spoken of the inevitable storms of life and the necessity of building our home on the foundation of Christ. How could we have ever imagined what our lives would be like less than four years later? A huge storm had swept over our home, threatening to take everything away; but by the grace of God, our little home was still there. I could not have been prouder of the family that remained.

Those days, grasping at normalcy or reminiscing about the old life most often brought a cold reminder that things were not as they used to be. Sadness could often overshadow what were once celebratory occasions. But not that day. As we remembered our sacred vows of marriage, things were just as they were promised to be.

A few days later, I surprised Katherine with a weekend getaway back to Malibu. It would be her first overnight trip. She had no idea we were going, but that morning, she perfectly set up the weekend by dreamily wishing for some time away from the grind of rehab.

After her swallowing therapy session, I packed her in the car under the guise that her final therapy session of the day would be at home. We drove past the house, where my mom was waiting at the front door with James in her arms. I told a very confused Katherine to wave good-bye to James for the weekend. And we were off!

I pointed our car in that familiar westward direction. Though Friday afternoon traffic in LA is horrendous, the momentary feeling of freedom together was the only thing on our minds. I turned on the CD mix I had made for our first joint birthday party three years before, held on our favorite beach in Malibu, "El Matador." We had carried a full spread of food and drink down a steep incline to set up this memorable event on the sand, only to have an unexpected rainstorm arrive along with the guests. And yet all our friends still came and ate and laughed and got soaked, and it was glorious.

Katherine asked, "Where is this song from? It sounds so familiar, but I can't remember how I know it."

As we turned onto Malibu Canyon and wound our way through the rugged mountains, that sentiment lingered. *Where are we? This place seems so familiar, like a dream just out of reach.* I silently prayed that this trip might be a cathartic and healing experience for us both, rather than a devastating return to our "old normal" before we were really ready for it.

A few miles from our destination, the road turned sharply and the view dramatically opened up, revealing the sparkling blue ocean. A bittersweet wave of memories flooded over us. Turning onto campus, with its manicured green lawns and warm terra-cotta-tiled roofs, its wild, grazing deer and the craggy hillsides tracing the sky, it seemed we had entered a place that had only existed in our minds. Suddenly I could recall the crisp smell of the eucalyptus tree outside our apartment window as easily as I could recall the sickly sweet smell of hospital anti-septic. This idyllic place would forever be memorialized as our first home together as a couple, yet it was also the place I packed up alone as Katherine lay hooked up to a life-support machine. It was where James came home from the hospital and where his mommy left home for the last time.

Katherine and I breathed in the scene and the memories deeply, and it hurt. We stayed at the campus hotel—no longer residents of this place, but visitors, spectators. One of our favorite spots at Pepperdine was nearby, a memorial garden honoring the victims of September 11. It offered an unobstructed vista, and a quiet stream flowed through its center, right into a still pool that overlooked the distant ocean. It felt holy there, like a natural cathedral memorializing many things lost and also whispering of many things yet to come.

From that vista, we could see the rooftop of the dorm we had called home—the place where we successfully cooked our first salmon with friends and then promptly dropped it on the floor, and where we deliriously struggled to put together a crib until the wee hours just days before James's arrival. Across the street from the dorm is the law school building where I attended classes for three years and stared at the same ocean view from the library while pulling all-nighters before finals. Below that, we could see the mailroom where Katherine was on a first-name basis with the postman, as she loved sending out copious amounts of letters. Farther down the hill was the track where we walked and talked about our future on gorgeous summer evenings. I could still see Katherine's pregnant silhouette fading as the sun dipped below the horizon. Just below the track was the pool where we took James to swim for the first time on a Friday night before everything changed. After getting out of the pool that night, Katherine had said she felt really strange, dizzy, but then the feeling passed. We thought she was having an odd reaction to the chlorine.

We left the garden by a side entry that was flat and accessible for wheelchairs, one we had never taken before. The words to Psalm 23 were etched on a series of stones laid down on the path. Like a well-worn hymn, those words were undoubtedly rolled right over by many, but that time, the path and the words came to meet us: "The Lord is my shepherd; I shall not want." The wheels of Katherine's chair clicked along the uneven places, reminding us of her mode of transport. Despite our disabilities and constraints, God had made a way for us to experience that moment—a moment we shouldn't be experiencing at all.

"He makes me to lie down in green pastures; He leads me beside the still waters. He restores my soul." We stopped for a moment, the prayers of the past months ringing in our ears, prayers for healing and restoration of body and soul. "Yea, though I walk through the valley of the shadow of death, I will fear no evil; for You are with me. Your rod and Your staff, they comfort me." We had brushed against death and grieved loss more than most people our age, yet as we stood atop the mountain and looked down on a life that might have been, we felt inexplicably comforted. "You prepare a table before me in the presence of my enemies; You anoint my head with oil; my cup runs over." The sea grass by the path moved as if it were waves. Against all odds, we were being filled up with hope—a hope that was overflowing onto others in need. "Surely goodness and mercy shall follow me all the days of my life; and I will dwell in the house of the Lord forever."

We went down to the beach at dusk before the purple and gold hues of sunset bled into the black horizon of the sea. The rhythm of the waves calmed our spirits. I hadn't considered that Katherine's wheelchair wouldn't work on sand, so we slowly walked together the twenty yards to the water's edge, one of my arms around Katherine and one laden with a blanket and bags of takeout from all our Malibu favorites: Greek food from Taverna Tony and Thai food from Cholada and a large slice of chocolate cake from Marmalade Café. Katherine couldn't eat any of it, but she just wanted to touch them to her tongue for a moment before spitting them out into the sand. I only complied because I felt this might be motivating for her next round of swallowing therapy on Monday.

The sand proved to be tough terrain for Katherine's shaken sense of balance, and the walk had winded her greatly. We sat in silence for a while, taking in this place through new eyes. She tasted a few of her favorites, her smile quickly fading as she remembered she could not really eat them. Her G-tube hung conspicuously from her stomach to the beach blanket. I poured her liquid dinner into the tube, filling her stomach but not her deepest appetites.

Like salt water to an open wound, this visit to the ocean was healing our past, yet each lapping of the waves stung like fire. As the last ember of light was extinguished in the water, we hobbled back to the wheelchair in near darkness, laughing at the sad spectacle we must be to the surfers and lovers sharing that stretch of sand. Against all odds, we had returned to these waters, and in so doing, we bolstered our resolve to return to them again.

Katherine

On the day before Thanksgiving, Jay rolled me into the radiology lab to take my ninth swallowing test. My in-laws were in town for the holiday, and I prayed we would soon be giving God all the glory, with big ole turkey legs and a pound of stuffing on my plate. My swallowing therapist fed me a spoonful of pudding while a moving X-ray of my head and neck was projected above me. I swallowed with all my strength, quite sure that Thanksgiving, my favorite holiday, was of course the most perfectly timed day for God to allow me to eat again. I was almost shocked when my therapist shook her head no, with a frowning downward gaze.

I wiped away tears of sadness, embarrassment, anger, and exhaustion as Jay dutifully pushed me back to the house and got me set up in the back of the living room. I can remember feeling so hopeless and helpless as I sat in my wheelchair observing the holiday "celebration." Despair washed over me as I watched Jay and his sisters playing with James, lifting him in the air and running around with him in circles, laughing out loud, while I could barely even hold my head up because my neck wasn't strong enough yet.

I found myself wondering, *Has God made a mistake? Should I have died? I'm caught between life and death. I can't even walk or eat or play with my child. I've gone from making lasagna in my little kitchen to being fed all meals through a tube in my stomach. I've gone from going on playdates with girlfriends to attending courses on disability adjustment. I used to power walk the hills of Pepperdine; now I have two physical therapists and a walker while I agonize to walk one step. I've gone from wearing a cute outfit every day to wearing adult diapers and hospital gowns. I want my old life back! But every day, that old life seems further and further away. If I weren't here anymore, things would be better for everyone. Jay could marry a normal, able-bodied woman, and James could have a normal mommy. Everyone could stop putting life on hold to help me get well. It isn't working. It isn't ever going to work. Jay and James and our sweet families don't deserve this suffering. I should be in heaven right now. Then at least everyone's pain would eventually come to an end.*

And then suddenly, before those thoughts had even fully landed in my head and heart, I felt a deep awakening of the Word of God, which I had known since I was a little girl. I could almost hear this rapid-fire succession of the truths of Scripture, like a dispatch from God Himself.

> *Katherine, you are not a mistake. I DON'T MAKE MISTAKES. I know better than you know. I'm God, and you're not. Remember that you were fearfully and wonderfully made in your mother's womb, and that is when the AVM formed in your brain.*
>
> *There is purpose in all of this. Just wait. You'll see. There is no replacing you! Jay could never, ever marry a woman as amazing as you. James could never have a mommy like you. Think about what this will mean for his life. Mommy's stroke will always be a part of his story. That is a gift to him. It will inform his life. Let him consider it pure joy as he grows. All of this will teach him in ways beyond anything you could say or do.*
>
> *Trust Me. I am working out EVERYTHING for your good. Don't doubt this truth just because you are in darkness now. What's true in the light is true in the dark.*
>
> *I know you can't fight this. That doesn't matter. All you have to do is be still and let Me fight for you. I will complete the good work I began when I gave you new life. I will carry it on to completion. Believe that. My*

nature is to redeem and restore and strengthen. This terrible season will come to an end. You will suffer for a little while, and then I will carry you out of this.

You will see My goodness in the land of the living. Lean into this hope. Let it teach you how special you are. Most people will never go through this kind of hell on earth. I have chosen you. Live a life worthy of this special calling you have received.

Something supernatural occurred in those moments as those truths hit me hard. God met me in the midst of the messiness of my life, and I felt fresh determination to press on and persevere. I suddenly felt extraordinary—in spite of my terrible pain. That moment changed everything for me. It was my epiphany of hope. I knew deep inside that my "earth suit" was only temporary. I would never lose heart in this situation because my soul was not what was wasting away. My body didn't work. That was all.*

From that moment, and slowly, one day at a time, Jay and I were learning not to hang out in the place of fear and of questioning what might happen.

There is something profound about hope, something so meaningful when you cling to what is beyond anything you know and understand. When that happens deep in your head and in your heart, something shifts. *Hope heals.*

When we arrived at Casa Colina, we were told that the average stay was sixty days. I had been approved by insurance for more than double that time already, so we had no idea what the new year would bring. I did know I needed a break from that

_____

* For a list of the Scripture verses that Katherine is referring to here, go to the back of the book.

place, though. The routine was exhausting and depressing, so I was elated when I was approved to take a two-week vacation to Georgia and Alabama for Christmas/New Year's and my sister-in-law Sarah's wedding. We were going home!

Thankfully, airline travel is usually made easier for people in wheelchairs, including shorter lines, preboarding, and bulkhead seating. It was almost fun to travel in a wheelchair. Almost. The flight home was magical to me after enduring all the hospitals and rehabs. F R E E D O M was exhilarating!

Jay went to the bathroom midflight, and I was left alone in our two-person section. A flight attendant approached me while he was gone. "Would you like a cookie, nuts, or pretzels?"

What? Would I like these? Well, YES!

Over the past eight months, no one had offered me food, much less asked about my preference for a salty or sweet snack.

"Cookies, please," I answered instantly. Always a sweets hound, nothing had changed in that department since April 21. I was not even thinking about how I would actually eat those cookies.

As the flight attendant handed me the package, I rabidly tore it open and tossed half a cookie in my mouth. Chewing quickly and then "swallowing" rapidly, I guess I knew on some level that this was not okay to be doing. Of course, the cookie came right back up, and I had to spit it into a napkin after repeatedly trying to swallow it.

Oh well, at least I got to taste a cookie. Jay—or anybody else for that matter—will never know about this eating attempt. I'm pretty sneaky.

When Jay came back to his seat, he instantly broke into a sweat.

"What's on your face? Is that food? Were you trying to eat something?" he said in a tone that approached a yell.

"What are you talking about? How was the bathroom?" I tried to change the subject.

He wasn't buying it. "What is that? Bread or a cookie or something? Where did you get it?"

Unbeknownst to me, I had spit up some cookie on the right side of my mouth. Since I had no feeling on that side, I had no idea it had lingered after I had disposed of the napkin and wrapper—all the evidence. I was busted! But it was worth it.

When we got to Montgomery, we celebrated Sarah's marriage to Jeremiah in a beautiful winter wedding. Then we traveled to Athens to join our family for the holidays. As we pulled into my hometown, I began to notice yellow ribbons tied around trees and signs welcoming me home. Apparently, the former mayor, a family friend, had emailed all the members of the Chamber of Commerce to encourage this touching show of support. When we turned into our neighborhood, there was a group of around sixty people standing on the first corner. As we drove by, I saw they were holding signs and waving yellow ribbons in my honor, and I cried as I accepted these love offerings. I felt cherished by my sweet hometown and so grateful for my first happy holiday since my life had changed forever.

Our holiday break had been encouraging yet draining in many ways. In one sense, we strangely welcomed coming back to the simple therapy life, yet it only took a few hours to remember that we much preferred anything to the monotony and tragedy that was daily life at Casa Colina.

Upon our return, we heard a story that broke our hearts. We had befriended a lovely group of Spanish translators, who were as much a part of the TLC therapy culture as the therapists. Though they were not working with Katherine, they felt very maternal toward her and looked out for her.

One in particular, Lara, was especially kind and interested in our family and James. She approached us as we entered the gym, giving us both warm hugs, but as she pulled away, tears flooded her eyes. "What's wrong?" we both asked quizzically. She told us that over the holiday break, her son was home from college and got into a late-night altercation with a bouncer at a bar, who hit her son in the head with a small club. The blow hit a major artery, causing a massive brain hemorrhage. He died of his traumatic brain injuries. "My only comfort is that he does not have to suffer in a place like this," she wept. "Though he is not with me, he is not trapped in a brain-injured body. He is with God." We cried with our friend over her incredible loss.

We later found out from a therapist that a TLC patient had died over the holidays too—the same patient who had cursed at us a few months before, on our first day of therapy. This was the third death of a fellow patient since we had arrived at Casa Colina, but it was certainly not getting any easier. One man abruptly died of a heart attack in the gym as horrified patients witnessed frantic therapists trying to resuscitate him to no avail. The other death, perhaps more merciful, came to a longtime vegetative patient—a decorated police officer hit by a car in the line of duty. He was a fixture of the TLC, a bitter-sweet reminder to us of our new peer group as he reclined in his wheelchair in the common area every day—until one day, when he was not there anymore.

Loss came in forms other than death as well. Susan was a fellow patient who had become a friend in the months of co-laboring in therapy. She had suffered permanent injuries to her body and brain from a car accident when she was in high school. Like Katherine's, her body was greatly impaired, but her cognitive abilities were intact. The two of them would commiserate about their unique struggles, and Susan gravitated to our family, as her own family was not around. After more than a decade of caring for their adult daughter, it seemed her family was no longer able to dedicate themselves to her profound needs. We wondered why we hadn't yet seen Susan since we returned from the holidays. We were told she had been transitioned to a long-term care facility, a nursing home, where she would live out the rest of her days. She was thirty-four.

During this same time, we finally visited a hearing special-ist, as this particular deficit had been relatively low on the triage list thus far. Though Katherine clearly had right-ear hearing loss due to auditory nerve damage during her AVM surgery, we had never received a definitive diagnosis. Despite the seem-ing ubiquity of being "hard of hearing," this issue had actually proven to be one of the more stressful changes in our marriage and in Katherine's interactions with the rest of the world. Her already impaired communication abilities and distorted speech were now further strained in light of not being able to hear when other noises distracted her or to know where noises were coming from. Miscommunication was frequent; repetition of the simplest sentiments was required often; and patience was growing thin on all sides.

When the audiologist tested Katherine's hearing, we heard a diagnosis that should not have been surprising but was none-theless surprisingly painful to hear: Katherine was permanently deaf in her right ear. Sometimes obvious losses must first be named before they can be grieved, and the grief came quickly as she heard the word *deaf* in her hearing ear—now her only hearing ear.

Katherine began to weep. I think she had always held out hope that her hearing might somehow heal and return over time; now it was clear it would not. Even the most cutting-edge treatments of the day could not help hearing loss caused by nerve damage.

We were routinely presented with all manner of death and loss as matter-of-factly as our morning newspaper. One day, a patient was struggling to recover his or her life; the next day, the struggle was abruptly over. One day, a long-hoped-for goal was revealed to be a dead end. Death with a capital "D" was present at times, but on a daily basis there were little deaths—losses that chipped away at our lives. Yet brain rehab is just an exaggerated picture of the knife's edge on which we all live every day. We assume too much about what our future will be like, based on what we have given and thus what we feel we are owed in return. And when this so-called agreement doesn't work out in our favor, when the gap between our expectations and reality is great, we feel cheated.

We began to recognize in our own hearts places where we were actually expecting more out of life and of recovery—better outcomes–than we were expecting out of God. As we intentionally and prayerfully offered up our fears, our purpose began to clarify. No matter what deaths, big or little, we would encounter in the year ahead, we felt empowered to live fully into this fragile existence with a newfound freedom, knowing that God would give us life in ways we could have never asked for or imagined.

Katherine

My twenty-seventh birthday was surreal. I was "celebrating" the fact that I had lived for another year, but my circumstances were heartbreaking. Nevertheless, I had been surrounded by love from the beginning of my ordeal. I was determined to enjoy my friends and family.

Everything at my birthday party was light blue, my very favorite color. All the guests and even baby James were dressed in blue. Before going to bed that night, we flipped through the pictures Jay had taken at the party—pictures of me in my wheelchair with James propped up on my lap, blowing out candles on a cake I could not eat, surrounded by friends and family doing everything for me because I could do nothing. Somehow seeing these visuals left me in a state of sad reflection. I still didn't even recognize myself in photos. And I still had so many questions I wanted to ask someone, anyone. For instance, *If I can't take care of my baby, what kind of mother am I? If I can't eat or speak or write normally, am I still a Southern belle? If I have no cycle, will I ever be able to have more babies?*

There were so many things the brain bleed had taken away, but the prospect of never bringing another life into the world was one of the saddest. Experiencing the beauty and joy of early motherhood with James made me want more babies. Obviously, right then would not be a good time to get pregnant, but at some point in the future, I wanted to have a lot more children. I told anyone who asked that I wanted four, five, maybe even six children down the road. As I faced what I expected would be a lifetime of limitation and sorrow, the reality of my losses hit me really hard.

I also realized more and more how much I'd taken for granted. Like driving the Pacific Coast Highway with all the windows down and the sunroof open. I loved the sense of freedom! Now I couldn't even get out of bed or go to the bathroom by myself. I wanted to get the remote that was just out of reach or tie my own shoes, but I knew I couldn't do it. The worst was when I would hear my baby crying and want to walk over to get him. In the moment, I'd forget I had no balance and was only focused on comforting him. It was horrible to remember I could not reach my own baby and soothe him.

Being able to walk was something I had certainly taken for granted. Now, not walking meant I had lost all ability to be independent. Without Jay behind me, even when I used my cane, I would fall immediately. If I were to fall on the kitchen floor, I would be there until someone picked me up. Getting the handicap decal for the car was also much more significant than

I realized it would be. Hasn't everyone wished they could park in those handicap spots sometimes? I had always wanted to pull into one at the mall or church or anywhere I was running late to. Now, parking in those spots made me feel miserable. While I was grateful to have the infamous decal because of the benefits it gave me, it was so sad that at twenty-seven, I had to use handicap privileges just to get around in the world.

My voice was still very weak and distorted. I had always believed that God would use my ability and love of public speaking for something, but how could He do that if I no longer had a voice? This was so hard to wrap my mind around. Before the stroke, I managed to use the most cell phone minutes per month of anyone I knew. I had talked to my grandmother in Georgia for about an hour every other day from the day I got married. I cherished that time and loved telling her everything that was going on with me. Now she could barely understand me. I'd even had a medical professional ask me if I was speaking English!

Much of the time, I felt like I was underwater, all by myself in a vast ocean. It was terrifying and freeing at the same time. It was terrible because I couldn't get out and was trapped and alone; yet there was a freedom under the waves of being responsible for nothing. Every decision was made for me while I drifted, feeling like I was just along for the ride. The problem was, my sweet baby and husband were above the surface, and it pained me as a mother and a wife. All I could do was tread water below while other kind souls took care of them.

Sometimes I just felt like God had hurt my feelings. I wanted to scream it: MY FEELINGS ARE HURT!

I was grateful to be alive for another birthday, but I was scared too. I was scared of not being able to walk, write, drive, smile, eat, or have babies again. I was scared of being in a wheelchair my whole life. I was scared of always being tired. I was scared of the future and scared of the past, and often I was terrified of my own life. I had faith, but I also had doubt. "Lord, I believe; help my unbelief" was a frequent prayer.

Much to my surprise, in the weeks following my birthday, I started to feel strangely okay. I was comforted by the dawning realization that I could choose what to do in this situation. It was my decision, the only thing I had control over. Even while feeling so powerless and trapped, I had this epiphany of hope. This terrible thing had happened to me, but now I would determine some things for a change. *We cannot control what happens to us in life, but we can control our reaction.* It may sound like a cliché, but it's true. In spite of the devastation of being made into this handicapped miracle girl, I determined to fight fire with fire. I could "be of good cheer," and I would "finish the race" set before me.

I kept hearing in my head the words to the old hymn "It Is Well with My Soul," written by Horatio Gates Spafford after four of his daughters drowned while crossing the Atlantic: "Whatever my lot, Thou hast taught me to say, it is well, it is well, with my soul." Truth be told, it *was* well with my soul. No matter my situation, no matter what was gone or missing, my soul could be well. Cultivating the simplicity of a childlike faith is often the most challenging task to take on, but when I really tried it, I found myself feeling more and more secure and at peace in my Father's arms.

After ten failed attempts, I was almost shocked when I finally passed the swallowing test, permitting me to eat some foods after eleven months without eating. I had always believed I would eat again someday, but when I was finally given the go-ahead, it felt like a dream, one made all the more astonishing when Jay informed me of the original prognosis that I would likely never swallow again. What a glorious moment when I heard, "Yeah, you can eat!"

Nonetheless, my new diet was not exactly an all-you-can-eat buffet. I was restricted to ten spoonfuls of thickened liquids per meal, and I could drink only carbonated liquids because the bubbles made the liquid thicker. I immediately started eating everything I could possibly swallow, including yogurt, Jell-O, baby food, Cream of Wheat, and mashed bananas! The different weights of these foods acted like dumbbells, strengthening my swallow, and their thick consistency made it easier for me to slowly and intentionally swallow them rather than risk having food slide into my airway accidentally.

I guess the swallowing therapist assumed I would use a normal-sized spoon, but my soup ladle definitely seemed to make the ten spoonfuls go much further. I wondered what might happen if I used a full day's worth of spoonfuls at breakfast. I decided I would just worry about that at lunch. I had an incredible breakfast my first morning: two bowls of baby oatmeal with cinnamon, a key lime pie yogurt, a glass of strawberry kefir, liquefied scrambled eggs, and a cup of thickened OJ!

Eating again was as phenomenal as one can imagine. The first time I tasted Jell-O again was one of the greatest days of my entire life. I was so happy that I sobbed. Jay and I spent close to $100 on every yogurt and Jell-O-like product we could find at the grocery store. We bought things I had never heard of, like panna cotta and mochi in a jar. Those next several weeks were filled with intense euphoria. I did not care that this diet was so limited or that it was only ten spoonfuls. I got to choose those ten delicious tastes, and I would treasure them!

One day, Jay pureed some piping-hot butternut squash and put a thick slab of butter on top. He added salt and pepper and a small amount of nutmeg. One tablespoonful *changed my life*! I was certain I had never tasted anything that delicious in twenty-seven years. It would be a while before I could eat the pizza, cheeseburgers, chips and salsa, sandwiches, and caramel cake I craved, and I would most likely not be able to eat any meat for a long time, but I was fine with being a vegetarian if it meant I could have something. Anything!

There was a domino effect from the food coming into my body. Eating—the most important thing on my wish list—was a huge catalyst to my progress, the beginning of everything else healing and changing for me.

With the perspective that the passage of time brings, I began processing my story, not only in my head, but with my family and friends. I even told one of my therapists of my desire to write a book about my experience and what I was learning. She replied, "All the patients here say they want to write a book, but the reality is, life after brain rehab doesn't usually allow for that kind of thing. Katherine, you be the one to do it."

Motivated by her words, I began to write down my story. I would often stay up late at night, pecking away on my laptop with my one working hand. In writing the details of what had happened, I began to deeply connect the dots of all the ways God had been working. This became my gratitude manifesto of sorts, and this practice of remembering began to change the way I felt about my current state and about my future. I wrote these words near the one-year anniversary of my stroke.

A year has passed since I almost died. I still did not begin to know everything about why this happened to me, but I did not believe in happenstance. I am convinced there are no mistakes and nothing is wasted. Several months before my stroke, I even mentioned to friends that I felt

God was preparing me for a change when James reached six months. In a weird way, it was as if I knew this was going to happen.

In spite of the fact that I am still pretty bad off, I can acknowledge the many, many miracles that have kept me alive and healing. I had a severe brain hemorrhage, the location and size of which almost always result in death or worse. I lived. My husband unexpectedly came home for lunch right before I collapsed and happened to be home to call an ambulance and be there for our six-month-old baby. I was taken to the UCLA Medical Center, which happened to be the third-best hospital in the country. Dr. Nestor Gonzales performed my brain surgery and he just happened to be double board certified in vascular neurosurgery and radiology. My husband just happened to take out a PPO catastrophic insurance policy for us more than three years before, without which we would have been financially devastated because of my injury. I happened to win $50,000 on a game show, and that money enabled Jay to care for me full-time. Our families happened to be willing and able to live bicoastally to help care for us, including my sister-in-law Sarah, who moved from Ethiopia to California, and my sister Grace, who chose to go to college in Los Angeles too. The worst thing happened at the very best time. Jay was almost finished with law school. I wonder what would have happened if it had been his first year. He was even allowed to graduate from law school between hospital runs. This also happened at the best time for our baby. What if he had been a newborn or a teenager, needing me more than at perhaps any other time?

I happened to speak about the notion of identity to our treasured Young Marrieds group before this happened. Even then, I knew enough to know I needed my identity to be founded in something beyond myself. I had just happened to memorize more Scripture in the year before my stroke than I ever had before. I didn't know it was because I would not be able to read or write and would need to know the truth about who I really was and who God really was. I had joked with the women in my discipleship group that they needed to memorize Scripture in case they were put in prison. I just did not know then that a prison could be one's own body!

Because of all the physical therapy, I am in the best shape of my life. Because I have been incapable of taking care of my son, I have not changed a dirty diaper in a year! Since I am now eating but cannot walk, I have breakfast in bed every morning. Because I am severely underweight, I have to eat Sprinkles cupcakes and Stan's donuts to try to gain it back. Even though I cannot write, there are multiple websites dedicated to what is happening to me and my family. The two main sites have received well over one million hits in more than one hundred countries.

Did I wish this had never happened to me? Of course. But an earthly body is a mere tent, and there is a purpose behind what happened. I had once heard that if we pray for patience, God doesn't just give us patience; rather, He gives us opportunities to be patient. If we pray for courage, He gives us opportunities to be courageous. I had always prayed for more patience because I was so impatient. I had always wanted things done right now! When praying about having James, I had asked for courage. I had always been a wimp, and if you told me this was going to happen to me, I would not have believed I could have survived under such circumstances. But the result is that I am learning volumes about patience and courage. And I am beginning to praise God for what He

has done, what He is doing, and what He will continue
to do. I have come to realize that believing in God is not
possible without also believing God. He says He is my
hope and strength, and I am taking Him at His word.

Jay

Had it been nearly a year since life as we knew it had been turned upside down? So many events had torn lines of demarcation through our memories, making them easy to recall, as if they had happened yesterday. On the other hand, the monotonous drudgery of therapy made the past year feel as though it had stretched out over decades, like we were living in slow motion. Regardless, many new challenges lay ahead, including the decision that Katherine would undergo a particularly radical facial surgery at UCLA.

The facial paralysis was slowly pulling down her right eyelid and cheek and lip. The ramifications of a face no longer controlled by a brain run far deeper than vanity. A paralyzed face greatly affects speech, swallow, and eye exposure, so we decided to move forward with a potentially two-part procedure that would effectively rewire Katherine's facial nerve circuitry. This had to be done within about a year's time of the paralyzing event, as her right facial muscles would soon be irreparably atrophied and unusable. We scheduled the surgery for a few days after the one-year anniversary of the stroke.

We stayed in Katherine's mom's apartment in LA the weekend before the surgery, and it was a sweet time with family in town and reconnecting with our LA community. But Monday, the day of the surgery, came soon. Stepping into a voluntary surgery felt so different from undergoing an emergency procedure. The waiting is torturous with both, but clearly the planned one allows you to anticipate and worry even longer. And with the great amount of medical experience gained during the year, it was hard for me not to be tormented with realistic imaginings of what Katherine would be undergoing in the operating room. It felt like déjà vu to be in the waiting room again, and yet the comfort of community was steadfast too.

In this first-phase surgery, a nerve from the area near Katherine's ankle would be harvested and connected to her left, working facial nerve. This "extension cord" would then be tunneled across her upper lip, where it would begin to grow toward her right, nonfunctional facial muscle. It was stunning to consider that such medical techniques were available to her. We were so hopeful for positive outcomes of the surgery and how they might propel us back to some semblance of our old life, one without a paralyzed face and not eating solid foods; yet we would be reminded that no amount of surgery or therapy could return Katherine to the way she was before.

Katherine's doctors were extremely pleased with the results of the surgery. We were left underwhelmed. There had been a small chance that this surgery would do enough to innervate the lifeless muscles in her face, but now it appeared she might need the even more radical second-phase surgery in the future.

On a brighter side, since the surgery had not negatively affected Katherine's swallow and since she was progressing in her eating, the doctors had approved the removal of her G-tube. This necessary evil had sustained her life for nearly a year, but it was an awkward appendage, connecting the inside of her stomach to the outside world, bypassing the normal ingestion process. Though it could be covered or hidden under clothes, it would often slide out of the bottom of her shirt at inopportune times, reminding us of just how sick she was. I hoped that removing the foreign object from her body would perhaps also remove the constant reminders that she was still unable to function normally. Excitingly for Katherine, with its removal would come the delight of taking baths again, one of her favorite activities, as well as participating in pool therapy, which would most assuredly help her relearn to walk.

Though we were continuing to notice a pattern of our miracles occurring in progressive steps, it was still hard not to yearn for quick resolution, and this yearning sometimes drew us away from common sense. Once the gastroenterologist had pulled out the tube in a swift and disturbing pop, we were emboldened to venture to the nearest fast-food joint for a breakfast sandwich, which was, admittedly, not on Katherine's currently prescribed diet of yogurts and thickened liquids. Freedom from the tube somehow meant freedom from reality. It was a nod to the road-trip fare of our childhoods, which were always associated with carefree, happy memories, and we sought to relive such feelings as we ravenously ate our sausage biscuits.

It took only a few seconds for Katherine to begin gasping for air and then cough hard but soundlessly. I beat her on the back until she wretched up the uncooperative remnants of biscuit and sausage. We looked at each other bashfully, ashamedly, stupidly. And we both began to cry, first out of fear, then out of anger, and finally out of relief. We pulled out of the parking lot, running over the cursed biscuit wrapper as we left, and headed back to Casa Colina for Katherine's first pool therapy session, which would be followed by a long, hot bath.

In conjunction with Katherine's latest surgery, our friends in LA wanted to show their support with a celebration of Katherine's life, which would also raise funds to help pay for the tens of thousands of dollars in medical bills we had racked up. It was humbling to accept such a gift, but we reluctantly did. It seemed so much had already been made of our situation, but our community wanted the best for us and didn't know how else to help.

They threw a "Katherine Lived" party, a wine-tasting/silent auction/live music event at a friend's spectacular home in the hills above Los Angeles. It was lovely in every way. We thanked the crowd, and Katherine even took a death-defying step with no cane as her high-heeled therapist spotted her confidently. The crowd burst into uproarious applause as if a gymnast just nailed an impossible landing. For many who had not seen Katherine since her stroke, it was an awe-inspiring moment to see the fruit of a year's worth of prayers. And yet, there was a sadness that lingered, a shadow that covered the celebration. Katherine was indeed there, but not in a state that anyone thought she ever would be in. As time passed and many deficits remained, it was easy to lose sight of the first major miracle—the new birth, the second chance to live again.

Katherine and I were regularly challenged by an unspoken question: *Would we still be able to thank God for what He had given, for what He had allowed to be taken away, and for what He had allowed to remain?*

The call to give thanks, not at the end, but in the midst, began to reverberate inside us. We may never arrive at the ending we hoped for, so if we waited until then to celebrate all that had been given to us, that celebration might never come at all. We were learning, ever so slowly, the truth of what John Newton wrote: "All shall work together for good; everything is needful that He sends; nothing can be needful that He withholds."

We decided that we would always celebrate April 22 as a reminder of the simple fact that "Katherine Lived"—that no matter what other things happened or didn't happen, there was a singular event that allowed her story to continue, an event always worthy of celebration and thanksgiving.

Katherine

One of the very hardest adjustments in my disabled body was the lack of coordination in my right hand. My brain could not seem to get the message that it could no longer coordinate fine-motor movements. Easily picking up and putting down objects, using my hand to brush my hair or apply makeup, handwriting, and even pushing my own wheelchair were terrible losses, and I was determined to overcome them.

In occupational therapy, my therapists would teach me how to use that messed-up hand for what they referred to as ADLs (Activities of Daily Living), which would eventually help me to do many of the things I had done with that hand before the stroke, but just to do it using other neural pathways in my brain. During that time, I did not understand that my messed-up hand was permanent. I thought it just needed to be "rehabbed" in the same way that my swallow had. I was (fairly) easily able to adjust to using my left hand for many tasks, mainly because I knew the change was temporary. While everything required more fore-thought, I knew that my right hand would work normally again one day and that this was just a period of adjustment.

Mother's Day 2009 was quite possibly one of the worst days of my entire life. Having completely missed my first Mother's Day in ICU, I wanted to relish my sweet son's presence with his mommy this year. While holding him during the festivities, I tried to reach over him with my right hand and accidentally hit him in the face. He sobbed and I sobbed while my mother, sisters, and Jay tried to console us both. I decided that moments of "normalcy" were not worth this tragic risk, and I resolved to back off from holding him until my hand worked normally again.

I harassed my occupational therapists and techs daily about my hand and the lack of coordination on my right side in general. I asked them when my hand would "come back" and "start working like it used to." I will never forget when I was finally told my hand/coordination would not "come back." This loss was permanent. I could not fully process that information. Right up there with my longing to eat and walk, I had a deep desire for my hand to heal. It would not be possible.

After that heavy blow, I was determined to get as strong as possible so I could compensate for the messed-up hand by my Wonder Woman-like strength and agility. In physical therapy, I would always ask for more exercises, do extra repetitions of any and every exercise I was assigned, and be the last patient to leave the gym. The therapists used a weighted ball in my sessions so I could practice carrying James around the house. Nicknamed "James the Ball," it became a legend around our gym. Eventually, it had stickers and a large blue label identifying him to the world. When training with "James," I would use my abdominal muscles to control my hand/arm and weigh it down enough to regulate the movements. While very effective over time, it was grueling. I developed the best abs of my life! Had I not had a feeding tube hanging over them, I think I would have worn midriff-baring tops to therapy (well . . . maybe not).

Though physical therapy was working, I still could not walk on my own. I had learned to walk with a cane with someone holding my back or holding a security belt around my waist, but I could not walk independently. I spent many months pounding the pavement and walking laps in the pool. I imagine I had taken tens of thousands of steps before October 21, 2009— exactly eighteen months to the day of the stroke—when I first walked on my own again.

After an invigorating aqua therapy session, Jay and I went back to the house in high spirits. I decided to try to walk slowly with my four-pronged cane, without Jay steadying me from behind. To our amazement and delight, I walked all by myself! Appropriately, Jay turned on a peppy Top 40 "female independence" anthem as the soundtrack for the milestone. I tried to do a little dance but almost fell over, so I just stuck with the plain walking for the time being. I beamed as I triumphantly walked through each and every room of our little house.

I wasn't going to be running any marathons, but in this joyful moment of recovery, it almost felt like I could. It was the beginning of a new kind of independence—or at least a new feeling of independence. Even though I walked slowly and with an assistive device, suddenly I didn't feel as disabled anymore. I felt healed . . . almost.

Jay

As we gained more footing in this new version of our lives, the scales began to tip toward doing less therapy and spending more time with James and in our community. The therapists at Casa Colina created a schedule for Katherine that gave her a few days off every week, making the most of her dwindling insurance benefits and reinvigorating her will to engage therapy more fully on the days she did go. On our off days, we would go to the local athletic club that had welcomed us graciously, and we would go to see movies and explore the quaint downtown area of Claremont, which had become a respite for us.

My cousin spent that summer of 2009 with us as a kind of companion for Katherine and James, as we had decided it was time for me to take the next step in my legal education and study for the infamous California bar exam. I had been out of the law school grind for a year, and instead of seamlessly moving into exam studies and taking the test a few months after graduation like my peers, I found myself in a very different scenario. While many of my law school friends were now jumping into new jobs, I had jumped into a totally different world. In light of the intense life-and-death conflicts I had personally encountered in the past year, I struggled to find purpose in revisiting something that now felt so unimportant. I think I resented the fact that many of my peers would consider the bar exam to be the pinnacle of their lives up to that point, the stress of which utterly overwhelmed many of them. I wished that the most stressful thing in my life could be a test. Nevertheless, I studied hard that summer, spending the bulk of my days at the local college library remembering how to read and write "legalese," poring over rules, cases, and logic. I took the test near the end of July and would not find out the results until November.

In that same season, anticipating a return to Los Angeles in the coming months, it had been brought to our attention that we just might have a home to begin our new life in. Amazingly, this potential home was the very one we had long dreamed of living in. Years before the stroke, some friends from our Young Marrieds group had stumbled on an up-and-coming area called Culver City and had rented a little yellow California bungalow right by City Hall. Culver City had a storied past as the location of a major movie studio in the early Hollywood days—filming classics like *The Wizard of Oz* and *Gone with the Wind*—and then sadly falling into disrepair and neglect. Only in the past twenty years had regentrification begun, enabling a little throwback small-town-USA to grow in the midst of the metroplex of Los Angeles. Two days before Katherine's stroke, she had hosted a baby shower in the yellow bungalow and had said to me how amazing it would be to live in that house and in that community someday.

Fast-forward a year and a half, and that house, actually a property consisting of three little bungalows squeezed together on a long lot, was coming up for sale, and, crazily enough, we felt compelled to try to buy it. Despite brain rehab and bar exams and unknown futures, we felt more strongly than ever that not only should we move back to Los Angeles, but we should figure out a way to make a home and a new life for ourselves in Culver City.

My father-in-law, who had worked in finance for his whole career, helped us secure the loan, and with the help of my family and some savings, we were able to buy this property we had only dreamed about owning. Since there were three houses, one would be ours, one would be for family members who would help us, and one would be rented out. The houses were tiny, one-level bungalows built around 1920. Our "big house" clocked in at around one thousand square feet. But the property felt like just the right place for us to start over. Katherine and James would, we hoped, be able to get around the house safely, and I would be able to manage the space easily.

We bought the property before it was even put on the market. Now we not only had a place to go after therapy, but we also had an embodied motivation, a vision to propel us through therapy into an exciting new season. We could hardly contain our joy.

As the fall of 2009 came to an end, we anticipated a return to the South for the holidays from Thanksgiving through New Year's Day. As we put together our Christmas cards between final sessions of therapy at Casa Colina, the anticipation of the holidays was palpable in a way we had never experienced before. Juxtaposed to Thanksgiving 2008 when Katherine could not eat and so much was still unknown, this season overflowed with so much promise, so much hope. We were being released from Casa Colina, a place that had given us miracles in terms of Katherine's recovery while simultaneously introducing us to one of the most challenging, painful experiences of our lives. We were grateful for it, but perhaps even more grateful to be moving on to something new.

I remembered with amazement the words of the admission counselor on our first day at Casa Colina: "The average stay here at the Transitional Living Center is sixty days." When all was said and done, Katherine had inexplicably been approved by insurance to stay in therapy for almost a year and a half. She had stayed longer than almost any other patient in the program, and the extended time had made all the difference in her recovery.

The day before we left for Thanksgiving, I received a letter from the California Bar Association that began with the line, "We regret to inform you . . ." I didn't need to read on. I had failed the bar exam after so much effort, not just on my part, but on the part of our families and Katherine, who had allowed me to step away from caregiving duties for a while to prepare. It felt like I had wasted those valuable months, all for nothing. I was now in a category that many law students find themselves in after years of education, loans, and expectations: I had failed the one test that mattered most. And yet in that moment, amid my disappointment and embarrassment, I knew there were tests that mattered far more than this one, tests I had passed. And I felt a peace, an assurance, that I could engage the holidays with joy and not shrouded in defeat. We would start a new year, 2010, in Culver City, in a new and beautiful life, and I would take this test again and pass it.

Nevertheless, the potential for hopelessness lingered even in the midst of the most positive self-talk, and the light at the end of the tunnel was still cloaked in darkness. Katherine had miraculously recovered but was still very, very broken, and now we were leaving the place that had helped her recover—and she wasn't completely fixed. Eating and walking had enlivened her in a whole new way, but I wondered how we would fare when the emergency mode of the past two years was finally behind us and the "new us" remained.

Amid the swirling fears of the unknown and the losses stacked higher than the victories, a question kept bubbling to the surface of my mind: *Will you trust Me still?* And I decided that no matter what lay ahead for us, we could not let anything obscure our view of the God who inexplicably gave us everything, even in the taking away. The God who gave us our deepest desires, not like a genie would, but like a loving Father who offers what we would want if we knew everything He knew. The God who ultimately gave us the one thing we needed more than anything else in the world . . . Himself.

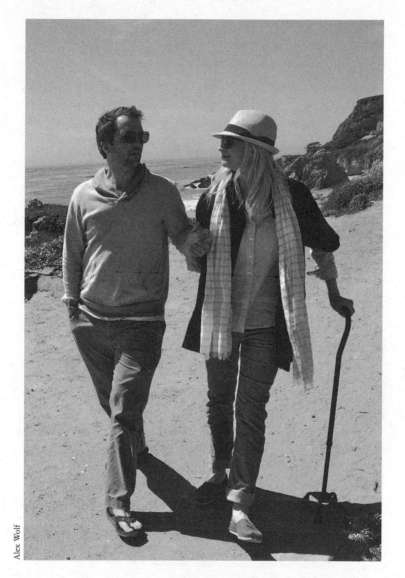

PART FOUR

Alex Wolf

THE HEALING
FOUND

Katherine

Before we could move into our house, we had to spend several days in a hotel while the house was being repainted and repaired. Jay worked there, just a few blocks away, while James and I mostly stayed put at the hotel. I cried more times than anyone would have imagined during those days. That hotel room felt like a reflection of my life. I was trapped, useless. Despite a deep desire to engage and help, I could not paint or unpack boxes. I hardly felt qualified to babysit my own child. Perhaps reality caught up with me all at once. I was starting to process the past year and a half, and ironically, the unwelcome visitors of bitterness and despair were settling into my heart just as I was finally coming home.

I don't think any of us can tell our most vulnerable stories in the moments they occur for fear that they may undo us. We have to wait until we are in a season of safety before we can open up our deepest wounds. This was mine: I had been to hell and back, with the scars and limp to prove it, and life had gone on for everyone else. What could I do with that?

Though we had shared openly with our digital audience during the time I spent in the hospital and in brain rehab, some of the hardest realities felt too raw to share publicly until much later. Perhaps like Mary after the birth of Jesus, I had needed to ponder these things in my heart, wrestle with them, and offer them to God before I offered them to anyone else.

The day before we moved into our bungalow, I decided to "speak" to whomever was out there on the web and wanted to listen. In early 2010, this was not as commonplace an occurrence as it is now. People usually didn't put deep feelings online and share stories of brokenness. For me, however, it was incredibly cathartic to click Publish, to put words to the deep groanings inside me, and in so doing, illuminate the darkest places and release some of the pain.

In a kind of stream-of-consciousness rant, like opening up a vein, I lamented about a number of topics that made me very sad as I reflected on my previous season of life. These seemingly disconnected moments of anguish popped like firecrackers in the night, each one sparking the next. I recounted stories that haunted me and posted a video I thought I would never show to my online audience because it was a more accurate physical representation of me than my readers could imagine by simply reading my writings—it was even subtitled because my spoken words were apparently that unintelligible.

Here are a few excerpts from that first post on February 2, 2010:

> There are really hard moments in this ordeal. Hard and depressing and heartbreaking and rough. Really rough. I could tell you story after story that would make you cry. It's been sad. You can imagine. Ironically, coming into a new season of physical calm does not always mean emotional calm. In fact, it often becomes the time and place when the floodgates open, and years of the darkest pent-up emotions overwhelm what would seemingly be a time of peace, even victory. Some of my deepest insecurities and fears have been exposed, and I am still trying to pick up the pieces of the dreams I had for my life—dreams that feel more like fantasies now. All my life, before the stroke, I had been confident, admired, and strong. I know in my head that I still am these things in many ways, but when your life is taken down to zero, it's hard not to feel that your ability to contribute as a human being is also zero . . .

Relearning to walk has been so hard. I have taken serious falls while under the care of many of the people who love me most in the world. One fall during a middle-of-the-night bathroom visit landed me in the emergency room at 3:00 a.m. I was fine, but I hit my head, and we don't take chances after the AVM. The pain of hitting my head paled in comparison to watching my guys sitting in yet another waiting room until the sun came up—all because of me . . .

July 13th of last year was such a sad day. James was taking a nap in his crib, and I was resting in our bed after a long day of therapy. The doors were open between the two bedrooms. Jay was at the front of the house, but within earshot if I needed anything. James woke up from his nap and said "Mama" clearly. It was the first time he had awoken and called for me in as long a time as I could remember. He wanted his mama to get him out of his crib, but his mama couldn't walk. I fought back sobs and said, as chipper as I could sound, "James, Mama can't come get you right now. Mama loves you so much, though." Then I dissolved into sobs. How could I live like this? What kind of mother can't get her baby up from a nap? I seriously considered just falling to the ground and crawling into his room, but I figured Jay would freak out. Even then, I still could not have gotten James out of the crib. Luckily, before I had time to consider other alternatives, Jay walked over and got James out. Ugh—it was so terrible. I will remember it until the day I die . . .

When I first viewed the video we shot last summer while my eye was still facing inward, I was so heartbroken. *Just look at me . . . Do I really look that way? Do I really sound that way? Ugh. My face, my voice—everything is just so sad. Do I really need subtitles now so people can understand my speech on video?* I guess in my pride I don't want people to know what bad shape I'm actually in. But this is reality. This is my reality now . . .

Strangely, I do not cry very much these days. A few weeks ago at our small group, however, I lost it badly. We were going around sharing prayer requests, and I started sobbing. I told them to pray for me because I feel like my life is on hold, in slow motion. Yes, I was alive and had recovered quite a bit, but I am still pretty bad off. Similar to my frozen face, my life feels frozen. Even though I'm OK, I still cannot function on my own. James may have to go to day care—which I have no problem with if a mom works, but I'm not working. I can't keep my balance, walk, read, write, eat, speak, smile, or live normally. Emotional scars remain. There is pain and stress and tension, and it wears on my relationship with Jay.

I cope with the sadness the only way I know how: I pray and ask others to pray. I simply don't know anything else to do. Don't think I'm some superspiritual person or have superhuman faith. I'm just in a really bad situation and need HOPE. Lots of hope. I am doing my best to "keep the faith." I heard recently that FAITH is an acronym for "Forsaking All, I Trust Him." And I do. I trust Him. I don't understand all this, and I don't pretend to, but I trust that there is a reason for this season of my life. I don't know much, but I know He is good, even when things are bad. And somehow, that's enough.

Much to my surprise, the response to my transparency was overwhelmingly positive. I received the largest number of comments on my websites I had ever received, dozens and dozens of emails, and countless handwritten cards from people all over the world. That post turned out to be the most shared and forwarded piece I had written so far.

That experience reminded me that vulnerability is contagious. When we share our stories in real and messy ways, we give people permission to do the same, and in the sharing, we release some of the things that keep us trapped in our own isolated hotel rooms. We remember we are not alone. And that brings hope.

Joy

We had long desired to move back to Los Angeles—to our community, to our people. It had been nearly a year and a half since we had gone to Casa Colina for therapy, and it had been nearly two years since everything had changed in our lives forever. Along with physical recovery, one of the great motivators during the endless months of therapy was the chance to return home. The opportunity to make a new life in Culver City was a stunning answer to prayer.

We were welcomed back with open arms, and it felt so good. We reengaged our church community, our small group, and our new neighborhood with childlike excitement. And yet it didn't take long to realize this transition would be almost as jarring as the one that followed the stroke. On one level, we knew things had changed; obviously, Katherine was very physically disabled, which limited everything we did. And yet, on another level, I think deep down we wanted to just tiptoe in the back door of our old lives and go about our normal business as if nothing had changed. It was soon apparent that such a course of action was not only a fantasy; it was impossible.

In the first few weeks after our return, we began going once again to our weekly small group. These seven couples had loved us so well in the aftermath of the stroke and would continue to in this new era. This intimate circle was a place of safety and support, an environment that gave us permission to let down our guards more and more, to grieve and hope among our friends. Many prayer times were spent weeping together, questioning how we might move forward in a world we were now acutely aware was not safe for any of us.

Our community was loving, concerned, and responsive; yet there was no denying that things were very different. Nearly our entire group of friends had gone from young married couples to growing families since our ordeal began. We were all in a period of transition, which made our acclimation all the more disorienting. It was hard for us to relate to the normal concerns of young family life after what we had seen and experienced. Lamenting sleepless nights, dirty diapers, and preschool applications felt like another language to us. We wanted to relate and engage because we were in that same life stage, but try as we might, we couldn't even fake it. Also, since Katherine no longer had her previous level of independence, nor did I, jumping in the car for a spontaneous playdate or meeting up with a group of people for a carefree dinner was not an option anymore. Over time, friends realized they would need to come to us, and they did; but in many cases, the invitations stopped, which we understood yet still mourned. It would prove to be less painful for us not to be invited rather than to try to reengage in ways that only highlighted the loss that was throbbing just below the surface.

Despite the struggle to find our bearings in our new life, we were finally getting back many of the most precious things that were lost in the stroke—Katherine's health, our community, a sense of home, and some autonomy in our adult lives. Deep gratitude flowed from our awareness that if only a few factors changed, our story would be completely different. What if we didn't have families who could help support us during this time? What if we didn't have insurance or financial resources?

What if we had nowhere to go? What if Katherine hadn't gotten any better?

And while digital community can never replace physical community, we were comforted to know that on the other side of our computers was a world of people hurting in similar ways. We began to sense new purpose and experience more healing as we were assured that we were not the only ones suffering. In sharing our pain, we were assuring others who were also isolated because of their physical limitations that they were not alone either. This virtual community became indispensable as we looked ahead to looming medical issues and struggles. Though we were now finally out of therapy, it seemed that the real, long-term work was just beginning. Katherine would require eye surgeries to protect the right eye compromised by its paralyzed lid and to hopefully correct her double vision. We were battling the insurance companies and hospitals, facing tens of thousands of dollars in contested bills, and we were denied home health help to allow Katherine to continue therapy at home.

These were not the normal concerns of your typical twenty-eight-year-old couple, and we felt alone in them. We found ourselves asking, *Is this what we hoped for during all those months away, all those months aching for home?* We became increasingly aware that when it seems you've gotten everything you hoped for and yet are *left* longing, perhaps those hoped-for things weren't the truest hope. If hope is only rooted in an outcome, then your expectations will crush you. This season of unrest began to spark a firestorm of questioning, and we found ourselves redefining many things in every area of our lives. *What was our truest home? What was our truest hope?* Could all the good things we longed for actually be drawing us away from the one thing that is the truest fulfillment of all our desires?

Katherine

Almost immediately after settling into our new home, I had a deep desire to get back into Bible study. I had participated in numerous studies and discipleship groups prior to my stroke. In fact, I was leading a women's discipleship group when I had the stroke. I recognized the tremendous benefits of these groups. Weekly, intentional accountability in life; "group therapy for Jesus" stuff; Scripture memory; disciplined time in the Word of God—all of this was part of what I had previously experienced and what I knew I needed to reintroduce into my current life and my struggles to ground myself in my new reality.

In March 2010, I decided to lead a Bible study on Esther by Bible teacher Beth Moore. I knew enough about Esther to know I wanted to study her after I'd gone through this terrible trauma. She was courageous, had some serious grit, and persevered through a nearly impossible situation. She proved to be a woman up for the challenge of her assignment in life. Yet she was also an imperfect and improbable heroine, one who struggled to find her true identity amid fear and isolation. I could certainly relate.

I gathered a small number of women to come to my home and do the nine-week study. We would watch a video teaching on each passage, and I would facilitate a discussion afterward. I knew that going deep into these teachings would be a lifeline for me as I began a new and difficult leg of my journey. Though God is never mentioned in Esther's story, His hand is evident in her circumstances, and I found it deeply encouraging to be reminded that God is always present, always working, even when it seems like He is not there at all. Revisiting the story of Esther in this particular season grew my faith in an unseen God and increased my patience in waiting for all He had done to be revealed one day.

My twenty-eighth birthday took place right around the time this study began. In contrast to the previous year, I was "in a good place," as the Californians say. As the Esther study unfolded weekly, I was finding my footing in the world again with things like truly happy birthdays and the joy of teaching and articulating the truths of the Bible through the lens of my new life experiences. Even with a severely disabled body, I could once again do many of the things I did before the stroke, and I finally felt like I was really living again, like I really had something to offer as a result of my pain. I would be lying if I said that all I'd been through was not terrible. It was worse than anything I could have ever, ever imagined. So much was different now, and it was really heartbreaking. However, I knew that nothing was stronger than God's power—a power that was at work in and through this broken vessel.

Near the end of Esther's story, a new phrase caught my attention, one I had never noticed before. These three simple words, "the reverse occurred" (Esther 9:1 ESV), seemed to be the theme of Esther's entire story—and perhaps the great theme of my story too. My life looked pretty much the opposite of what I had always thought it would, and yet God would take my crushed expectations and somehow make something better out of them—something that I could not even imagine. Yes, the reverse does occur in the kingdom of God. Perhaps the only greater reversal than a stroke might be the way in which God would heal me through it.

In true divine fashion—a "God wink" as I like to call such moments—the last night of the study was April 21, the second anniversary of my stroke. It seemed that God was preparing me for what was next: the next anniversary, the next hardship, the next joy, the next setback. This anniversary would always be a reminder of how my life had changed. However, now it would also be a reminder of all that God was continuing to do, not only in me, but also through me. I heard somewhere that challenges make you either bitter or beautiful (like Esther was, I suppose). Symbolically, with a face that was paralyzed on one side, I was choosing to be beautiful . . . gorgeous, in fact.

Jay

As I rolled over each morning, through the early light seeping in around the curtains I would stare in awe at the new woman who lay beside me. In many ways, Katherine was the same woman I had fallen in love with in the college cafeteria ten years before; and yet in just as many ways, through the refinement of suffering, she was a different person. I was different too, both inside and out. My newly graying hair belied my age. When people expressed surprise that I was not even thirty yet, I would tell them, "It's all the years of hard livin'."

Every marriage experiences the inevitable fading of the honeymoon period. Every married person is confronted with the reality that the one they married might be different from the one they thought they were committing to on their wedding day. This disenchantment, this space between expectations and changing realities, is often the beginning of the end of many marriages. But it doesn't have to be.

On our wedding day, I had no idea that, literally underneath her bridal veil, Katherine bore a microscopic abnormality, an AVM, that would forever alter the course of her future and mine. And yet this is a picture of marriage in the way that God fashioned it. When we get married, we manage to look the most attractive we will ever look in our lives, yet each of us bears much underneath the surface that will change that appeal—some things we already know about and some we could never imagine. This sounds hopeless in a way, like we're all marrying strangers; yet the reality is that marriage can bind our hearts together in an unconditional love that our human emotions could never manufacture on their own. Marriage invites us into a promise we may never have had the courage to make, had we known all we would be agreeing to. But rather than creating a prison—a "ball and chain"—marriage can provide a place of freedom, a garden of abundant life unleashed, in spite of all we did not know. When marriage is viewed in this transcendent way, though pain and sacrifice and loss still inevitably come, they no longer pose the same threat because the marriage, not the emotion, is the thing holding it all together.

There was no singular moment when I decided to stay in my marriage. It was more the accumulation of each day's choice to stay, of each day's intention to find awe and empathy and love for this woman who had been, quite literally, reborn. And yet in the physical staying it became clear that I would also need to commit to stay internally as well. What was my commitment worth if my body was in it but my heart was not? I was struck by the picture of God allowing people's hearts to harden, like the pharaoh's in the book of Exodus, or correspondingly to soften. I began to pray specifically, as in Ezekiel 11, for God to take away my heart of stone and give me a heart of flesh, one that was soft and tender toward my wife.

If suffering is like going through fire, I wanted to choose what this inescapable process purified in me and what it melted away. I found my faith and my hope solidifying into something more constant than my emotions or circumstances, creating an altogether separate organism—and that was so freeing. Similarly, the commitment I had made to my marriage was growing deeper, more enduring, and less dependent on whether a given day was a good or bad one.

Yet as the patient/caregiver routines became more entrenched in our lives, as the adrenaline left me and fatigue set in, I could see how that specific part of our relationship could be most rife for a hardening of my heart. As suffering does, this experience had pared away any pretense between us and homed in on our core issues, the core of who we were. Thankfully, as I had known all along, Katherine's core was pure, though her body and heart had been broken in so many ways. What was exposed was not bitterness or rage, but rather her abiding love. I prayed the same could be said of my core.

Nonetheless, when you put two very different, firstborn, achiever types in a relationship where they are supposed to be one, sparks will fly in both good and bad ways. When you layer on top of that the stress of life and death, the fear of the unknown, and the realities of severe disability, those sparks can light a fire that will either take the whole house down or melt away many imperfections, leaving something that just might last a very long time.

In our new home setting we felt safe, but in an unexpected way, the "honeymoon" phase after the stroke was fading, and we were both trying to embrace the new people who remained. Sometimes before bed, the stress and weariness of the day would induce an argument of one kind or another, but I knew Katherine still needed me, quite literally, more than I needed to be right. Still fuming, we would submit in that moment to care and to be cared for, not so much out of love for each other, but out of love for God and gratitude for the relationship He had given us—a relationship the whole of which was growing far greater than the sum of its individual parts. I would help Katherine to the bathroom and hold her chin in my hand while I flossed her teeth. She would lie down on the bed and I would gently begin the required nightly routine for her impaired eye, moisturizing it, putting in the lubrication, and then patching it shut with paper tape. There was no running out and slamming the door, going on a drive or sleeping on the couch. Yet in the humbling process of serving, even when I didn't feel like it, my heart once again softened toward her. I found that acting in love inevitably provoked true feelings of love, and the reverse was no less true. In the daily melting away of frustration and bitterness, we could embrace and celebrate the gift of this new life together, and in the midst of the mundane we could remember the miracle.

In light of my previous failed attempt to take the California bar exam while Katherine was in brain rehab, we decided the summer of 2010 might be the right time to try it again. If I had not already put so much into my legal education, with the passing of this test being the final leg of the journey, I probably would not have voluntarily entered into this hellishly stressful experience. Perhaps I wanted to justify my existence outside of being a caregiver, or maybe I wanted to justify the law school loans I would be paying until old age, but I think I needed to test my newfound confidence, my hard-won resilience, outside the walls of the hospital. I wanted to prove that my new self, born of suffering, might have something to offer the world.

My parents and in-laws were encouraging and supportive, orchestrating an elaborate schedule to temporarily unwind my now hardwired caregiving tendencies so I could fully focus on preparing for the test. Katherine and James would go on an adventure back South for a little more than a month while I prepared in California alone. It was a bittersweet decision, and I was confronted with the reality that Katherine's and James's futures, while inextricably linked to mine, were ultimately out of my hands. This was the first step of releasing—not releasing the attachment and the care, but releasing the illusion of control. As much as Katherine and James were my dependents, it was increasingly clear that we were all fellow dependents of God.

The weight of everyone's sacrifice was heavy at times, and I tried not to let the lengths to which everyone had gone add to my inevitable stress. Katherine was being stretched far outside of her normal comfort zone, but it seems such efforts always result in growth. In some ways, she had been kicked out of the nest for my benefit, yet in so doing, she was learning how to fly. My dad, the consummate pastor-encourager, was delighted to have a ministry buddy for part of the summer. He would carefully pack Katherine in the car and take her to visit nursing home residents or to share her story with a small church's congregation or on a local radio station. A few weeks of such packed scheduling took its toll on Katherine's still-frail constitution, yet it energized something deep inside her. She saw the impact that her suffering and her story had on people, not just in digital manifestations, but with real-life people, face-to-face. These were seeds of ministry planted in her heart. As a welcome counterbalance to the full schedule with my family, her parents gave her an equally needed opportunity to rest in the home of her childhood. It was restorative in a way that only one's original embodiment of home can be. All these goings-on helped encourage me that I wasn't wasting everyone's time and that perhaps there were greater purposes for all of us that summer than solely my test preparation.

In late July, I spent three days holed up at the regional California bar exam testing center with hundreds of other would-be attorneys. The weight of the expectations in that auditorium was unlike anything I have ever experienced, and yet this time, I did not feel like I would be imminently crushed; rather, I felt that regardless of my passing or failing, I would come out on the other side of this experience stronger. I felt more prepared than the last time, but perhaps less sure that I had a definitive role in the outcome. At some point during that summer, I think I released not only my control over the lives of my family but more of my control over my own life too. I was seeing that my most vital role, maybe my only role, was as a tool in God's hand. I was not the maker of my life or the writer of my story; God was—and that was a good thing.

Katherine

It seemed our new suffering personas were here to stay. We were *those* people now. The ones who had that thing happen to them that no one would wish on their worst enemy. People began to view us differently, set apart even. Our presence alone stirred many to a "carpe diem" fervor, while others felt deeply convicted, shamed, maybe even judged. We were seen as saints by many and likely as hypocrites by others. The experience of great loss and pain early in our lives had given us a strange and complicated position in relation to other people. I just wanted to be one of the girls enjoying and consoling my friends at the girls' night out, but those invitations dried up for a while. It took some time before our friends felt they could be vulnerable with us about what seemed like small disappointments in comparison to ours.

And truthfully, sometimes I wanted to scream from the mountaintops, "Your life's not that bad—stop whining!" while simultaneously cheering, "We did it. You can do it too!" Finding the balance between these two sentiments would prove far more difficult than we anticipated. It was tempting to think of our story as the baseline for hardship, the very definition of suffering. It was challenging to know how to embrace a role we never asked for. After leaving the perspective-inducing confines of brain rehab and then being surrounded by people and stories that were largely "normal," it was hard to battle the natural inclination to assume that the world revolved around us. We fought against annoyance and even resentment for the manufactured stress of our frenzied culture, for the constant hand-wringing over new parenthood, for the destructive patterns that seemed self-imposed, and for the overly dramatized problems born of narcissism and anxiety. Though we never voiced our annoyances, perhaps people picked up on them, or maybe they just assumed we could no longer hold a space for what felt like the trivialities of their lives.

It took time for us to find our place again in our community. We intentionally took on a leadership role in the Growing Families group at our church, and Jay even began hosting an early morning men's Bible study at our house. This reengagement was challenging but fueled by a newfound understanding of just how much we needed it all. As we began to see the universality of pain through the lenses of real lives and real losses, we became less inclined to view suffering as some sort of artificial hierarchy. We were receiving an increasing number of emails from people all over the world who were dealing with strokes or brain injuries, as well as many others who were dealing with cancer, divorce, betrayal, and the death of children. The stories inspired me and made me cry, but through daily interactions with our friends in the flesh, we came to understand that a person can justifiably be suffering, even if they are not in a life-and-death crisis, and we needed to validate that for those we were in relationship with. As we did, the way we were perceived and the way we perceived others began to change. More and more, we could see our story as a microcosm of everyone's story and our losses and gains as representative of the human experience. And we were recognizing the innate power in simply telling our story, both to inspire and to offer perspective. We began to see this dual role as part of our calling, flip sides of the same coin, to both encourage and awaken, to commiserate and motivate.

Naturally, our individual story will seem to be the central story in all of creation because in each of our tiny, personal universes, it is! But we are all in pain, though the sources vary. This understanding should inspire us to love everyone well, even when we feel we are the ones most hurting and thus most deserving of everyone else's attention and love. When we collectively mourn our losses and strain toward hope, our hearts expand. We begin to respond with empathy and realize that we all share the story of brokenness, and thus we all share the need for hope.

The initial cross-facial nerve transfer surgery I had in April 2009 lasted thirteen hours and was terribly painful and hard on every level. It was the first time I had voluntarily gone into surgery, and the waiting and the fear rivaled the intense pain. I prayed it would be the last surgery. But the doctors had told us there was a chance they would need to do a "phase two" surgery a year later to complete the facial reanimation. After much testing, it was determined that we would need to go ahead with this second surgery.

On September 17, 2010, I underwent a twelve-hour operation in hopes of giving new life to my lifeless face and eyelid and mouth. They literally took off the right half of my face. Then they took an inner thigh muscle from my left leg, transplanted it into my cheek, and connected it to the new nerve in my face from my first facial surgery.

I was in the hospital for more than a week, and Jay stayed by my bedside like a sentinel. The transplanted muscle was checked on every hour for days via a loud, buzzy sonogram machine that prevented rest of any kind. I had horrific ports in my neck draining excess fluid, as well as a "blood juice box" draining my inner thigh where the muscle had been removed. I felt like Frankenstein. In the midst of delirious pain and sleeplessness, I wondered, *Was it worth it?* My body was being dismantled, literally, in order to fix the broken parts.

This may well have been one of the very worst weeks of my life, but Jay and I tried to make the best of this terrible time. We binge-watched Netflix and ate donuts from a delicious shop nearby. We certainly didn't laugh much, but we didn't cry much either. It seemed that enduring such experiences was getting to be more commonplace for us, for better or for worse.

My parents kept James that week. During his first visit to see me, he took one look at my face, which undeniably was swollen to grotesque, pumpkin-like proportions, and said bluntly, "I wanna go home now." It nearly broke my heart. The same face he first stared into moments after he entered this world now scared him, and I felt ashamed. Jay helped wipe the tears from my bandaged cheek.

Our faces mean something, something much more than just beauty; they reflect our very souls to the world. All my life, I had greeted the world with a vivacious, toothy grin, and as a five-foot-ten blonde with big blue eyes, I didn't go unnoticed in many rooms. Yet now, though much of that had changed, ironically, I still didn't go unnoticed as Jay wheeled me into a crowd, my stature now slumped, along with half of my face. At this point, I didn't want my modeling career back, but I didn't want my child to run out of the room at the sight of me either.

Though the surgeons were extremely pleased with how the surgery had gone, we were again left underwhelmed. Were we looking in the same mirror as they were? Perhaps our expectations had been unrealistic, which is most often the case when life disappoints us. I suppose I thought—after so much effort and pain—that when I finally looked in the mirror again, I would see the same face I had always seen, the same one I had before the stroke. Months after the surgery, after all the stitches had been removed and the swelling had finally settled, I was left with my new face. Admittedly, the telltale droop of facial paralysis had greatly lessened and my face was actually pretty symmetrical at rest, but when I burst into a spontaneous smile or began to talk excitedly, it was clear that something was not right. It would take a long time before I felt comfortable with having my picture taken, and children would still inquire, "What happened to your face?"—and yet in my post-stroke existence, for better or for worse, a paralyzed face was far from my biggest problem.

I suppose more than anything I wanted to look in the mirror and see the real me staring back and be okay with her. Regardless of the surgery's outcome, regardless of who I had been or who I was becoming in the future, I began to make peace with the girl in the mirror, because that reflection was an accurate reflection of the soul within, battered but not broken, beautiful but not bitter.

Joy

In October 2010, we met with Dr. Gonzalez for an annual MRI and follow-up appointment. Katherine had a unique relationship with this neurosurgeon who had played such a vital role in saving her life. She was unconscious during most of the interactions early on, so to her, he was like a distant relative whom she felt she should know but only remembered hazily. I, on the other hand, burst into simultaneous smiles and tears at the sight of him, and we always shared a familial bear hug, as we had uniquely experienced coming so close to Katherine's death together. More than almost anyone in our lives, he understood just how far Katherine had come, and it moved him to anticipate just how much more improvement she might have.

Each year, we would bring with us a bottle of the nicest champagne we could find. What do you give a person who has given you something priceless? Almost every conceivable gift seems to fall woefully short of the object of its gratitude, yet this gesture was a simple nod that we celebrated and gave thanks for Katherine's life and for the man who had dedicated his own life to this calling so that his patients might regain theirs. The bottle sat on his desk, wrapped in a large gold bow, as we waited for him to enter.

When the door cracked open, I rose from my seat to greet him. As his gaze fell on us, his expression turned, not into a smile, but into a frown, and it seemed he might start crying. When your doctor starts the appointment with his own tears, you know it's not going to be a great experience for anyone. I sat back down quickly after a cursory greeting. He pulled up a stool and sat down right in front of us.

"There is good news, and there is bad news. In reviewing your most current MRI, I am glad to say there is no residual sign of the AVM that was removed or any other malformation in that area. The site of that surgery looks just right. However, Katherine, since your very first scans on the day of your stroke, we noticed and have been watching a totally separate neurological issue that we have not told you about yet."

The invisible gut punch landed. "Katherine, I'm so sorry, but you have an aneurysm behind your left eye."

This must be a mistake, I thought, *a misreading of the MRI.* But the look on Dr. Gonzalez's face let us know it was clearly no mistake. For a moment, as I looked at Katherine, now visibly deflated as she processed the news, I felt hurt, like a child realizing he had been left out of a conversation that directly affects him. *They knew this all along?* I saw the celebratory gold bow just over Dr. Gonzalez's shoulder, and it seemed so pitiful. "Cheers!" it seemed to shout out foolishly, like a late guest to a surprise party.

"Katherine, patients with a vascular malformation as large and complex as your AVM will often have a minor aneurysm associated with it. In the vast majority of these cases, 80 percent of the time, the aneurysm will go away within two years of the AVM removal. Each time we scanned your brain over these past two years, I so hoped this aneurysm would be gone, but it is not. I am so sorry."

Katherine began to tear up as she exhaled a sigh of confusion. This was clearly not the news we were anticipating for this routine checkup.

A barrage of questions began to well up in me. *Could the aneurysm rupture? What would happen if it did? Can you help us?* I needed to understand this problem so we could go about systematically weighing our options and fix it.

"The aneurysm is small, with a relatively low risk of rupture in the next five years. It is located in the internal carotid artery—the carotid cave—just behind your left eye." This revelation made me choke up as we had spent much of the past year focusing on Katherine's eyes through multiple surgeries seeking to protect her impaired right eye and also seeking to remedy the double vision she silently suffered with every day. If this aneurysm was behind her left eye, her "good" eye, then it seemed this aneurysm also put her vision at risk. The gut punches had turned into kicks.

My ire and hurt turned to God. *I thought we had a deal!* I wanted to scream. Two years after the stroke, we were coming to a place of peace regarding the suffering God had allowed us to experience. As Katherine recovered and we settled into a new life, we were finding hope in who God is and who He would be in the midst of our pain. Yet this moment revealed the invisible fine print I had tacked on to our "agreement" with God moving forward. It read something like this: *Due to the extreme nature of our suffering, especially at such a young age, the quota on suffering in our lives has been met, and* **no further suffering will be required.** While the aftereffects of suffering from the stroke might reasonably continue, I was sure it would not be reasonable for God to allow suffering to occur in other areas of our lives. And it went without saying that in terms of future suffering, the brain was totally off-limits.

Seeing that we were reeling with the news, Dr. Gonzalez assured us. "I want you to remember that aneurysms are my specialty, and decades ago the UCLA Medical Center actually pioneered the most highly regarded, least invasive technique for aneurysm removal." These tidbits were strangely comforting. After all, two years ago we didn't even know UCLA had a hospital, but this place and this team had changed the course of our lives. Now it was clear that our relationship was far from over. For a place to embody many of the worst and best moments of your life is bizarre and bittersweet, yet one thing was clear: If we had to endure so many medical challenges, we wanted to do it there.

The doctor continued. "I am so sorry to have to tell you this news, but I want you to know that the chances of it rupturing are so low that in my opinion the best course of action for now is to simply monitor it for growth on an annual basis."

In moments of great stress, it is advisable not to make big decisions and thus necessary to enlist the most trusted wisdom you can find. We trusted Dr. Gonzalez now in the same way that we entrusted Katherine's life to him years before. We felt his empathy for us. It was clear he hated this reality almost as much as we did.

We left that day with tearful, quiet hugs. I pointed sheepishly to our celebratory thank-you gift on his desk, and his earnest nod acknowledged the gift's irony as well as his thanks. And yet, maybe it wasn't as ironic and pathetic as it felt. Maybe it was actually the most important kind of gift for that kind of moment because it represented our gratitude for all that our friend had done and a "thank you in advance" for all he would do. Conditional gratitude is not gratitude at all. Real gratitude draws us into a celebration of thanks in the midst of doubts and fears—and not just in spite of them but because of them. We could celebrate our friend, celebrate who God had been and is and will be, and celebrate this life, even one with an aneurysm, because we knew it was all a gift, and we knew the Giver.

As we sat with this development in the subsequent weeks, a message became clearer: We were still here for a reason. There was still work to be done. God had never promised us an end to our struggles—not on this earth. As much as we longed for an end to the pain, as much as we wanted to cling to some artificial agreement that would give us a pass or a privilege because of all we had endured, we knew to do so was not only fruitless but missed the point. Did we want what He gives or did we want Him? Did we want the deliverance from the hurt or did we want the Deliverer of hope?

God was inviting us into a deeper relationship with Him. He was inviting us into a relationship of trust, built not on what He would give us but on who He was.

Katherine

In spite of receiving the shocking news of the aneurysm, we actually had a really wonderful autumn. James started pre-school in September, and each week just got better and better as our sweet little man thrived in that classroom setting. Even if his mommy was in a wheelchair now and his earlier days had been spent in hospitals and rehabs, he could go to preschool and play and just be an average kid. I felt like a "normal" mommy too (whatever that means). I loved his preschool and cherished how they took care of our little family.

Jay found out he passed the California bar exam, and we thanked God for this incredible milestone in our lives. He was now a bar-certified California attorney. This was an amazing accomplishment for anyone. Considering the past two years of our lives and his failed attempt the year before, this was like Christmas come early for the Wolfs! He would soon begin doing some legal work from home, consulting for various businesses while taking care of James and me. We were back from hell, and it was time to party!

We were getting more comfortable in the discomfort of our new life after a full year of living in Culver City. We were finding our place again. This season was full of celebrating community, of opening our home and dinner table, getting to know new faces, and reconnecting to old ones. There were parties and dreams and outdoor brunches and impromptu road trips and James—our sweet baby James. Paralleling these blessings were multiple eye surgeries; bad falls even in our tiny, one-story house; ongoing therapy and occasional breakdowns; insurance disputes; and the growing up of our baby much too quickly. Nevertheless, we chose to celebrate all the good rather than dwell on the broken.

Toward year's end, we traveled back South where we were scheduled to speak for the weekly chapel service at our alma mater, Samford University. We shared our story of what had happened to us *only four short years* after we had sat in that very same chapel and met on that very same campus.

The students were in awe. We could be them. We *were* them. We felt deeply privileged to pass on the truths that had gotten us through our ordeal, and we were delighted to share what had kept our young marriage together during those dark days. It was a beautiful, full-circle moment to be able to pass on wisdom from our journey, a journey that had started in that place.

We ended the year with what was one of the most fascinating occurrences that God had orchestrated post-stroke. CNN did a piece on our family at the very end of December, which aired multiple times from December 21 to 26. It was significant and symbolic to us that God's miracle in our lives was first showcased to a large audience throughout the holiday week. A true Christmas miracle was documented and seen by thousands of people.

We felt such a sense of purpose in sharing our journey. It was energizing and life-giving to impact others through our story of suffering. We were coming to understand more and more deeply that the stories that have the greatest impact are the ones that are hard, painful, gritty, and real—and more often than not, ones we never would have chosen for ourselves. We knew there would likely be more pain ahead for us, but the opportunity to inspire others became a reason to get out of bed in the morning into a world and a life we never could have imagined.

Joy

In spite of our struggles, we were experiencing some profoundly joyful times, and it was beautiful to see the synergistic quality of joy and sorrow intertwined. The more deeply we experienced one, the more deeply we could experience the other. We began to visualize this dichotomy as living wholeheartedly but with open hands. The choice to simultaneously live abundantly while releasing control strained all our seams at times, but we were learning that we could not receive anything when our hands were tightly gripped, even on the things that were most precious to us.

One night, I decided to sort through photos from before and after the stroke and tuck them into the frame of a large mirror in our house. It was a full-body mirror, one we used daily. It seemed appropriate to have the reflection of our present-day selves be surrounded by this photographic halo of memories—of moments of sweetness and reminders of loss. A shot of pre-stroke Katherine devouring a cupcake next to a picture of her empty ICU bed profoundly communicated the poignancy of this mix of joy and sorrow more than words could muster. As we looked at ourselves in that mirror, surrounded by the photographic stories of our lives, we knew that the removal of even one photo, one story, would change everything for the people reflected there.

One day, in the summer of 2011, as I was helping Katherine out of the bathtub, she excitedly told me she had just done some amazing thinking while bathing and had settled on a new direction for sharing our story. For years, we had been sharing on a website called katherinewolf.info, the same site where prayers and updates had been posted immediately following Katherine's stroke, but now we were feeling called to continue sharing our story through a more universal lens. Rather than just being an outlet for our very specific situation, we wanted to share more general encouragement with a broader audience.

"We should call our new website 'Hope Heals,'" Katherine said excitedly. "You know, like in Hebrews 6:19 where it says that hope anchors the soul. Anchoring in Jesus is the thing that heals our souls, and our souls are where we need the most healing anyway!"

This was the beginning of a new website, a new leaf we could float out into the digital stream. Our calls to action were summed up in mantras like "too blessed to be bitter," "don't wait to celebrate," "hope while you cope," and "heal in your home." These helped communicate the hard-won truth of what we were learning—that spiritual healing is the most important healing we can ever receive, and the means through which we might find that healing is through Jesus Christ—what He had done, is doing, and would keep doing for us.

As we entered a new season with a renewed vision for our life calling, we took some measured risks, delighting in what God was inspiring in us rather than allowing the fear of what we had experienced and what we might experience dictate how we lived. Katherine rarely ventured outside the nest of our home without me, but she joined Community Bible Study, a multi-generational gathering with a fantastic kids program. Every

Thursday, I would help her and James get ready, and some friend who was also attending would pick them up. The picture of them holding hands as they waited by the front door for their big weekly outing made me smile. Though there was always a fear of what might happen outside my protective arms, I knew Katherine needed to feel competent and independent again. She had been forced to resign so much of her motherhood, and helping her reinstate that role was one of my life goals.

In that same season, we also began planning our first international trip since the stroke. This was a significant milestone, as travel had always been a hugely influential part of both our pasts, but its appeal had faded in light of the obstacles of disability. For us to even consider such a trip signified great healing, not only of body, but of our desire to risk—to jump into an unsafe, unknown world and explore it with delight.

In celebration of our joint thirtieth birthdays, we decided to go to Italy (oh, and because we had a free place to stay). There was great excitement in the planning, and we cobbled together credit card points for the flights—one benefit of having a large amount of medical bills—and researched rental cars that could fit a wheelchair in the back. I wasn't about to try to drive a stick shift on the one-way cobblestone alleys of the ancient Umbrian city of Amelia where we would be staying, but the only available automatic transmission car was so small it looked like a team of clowns might come honking out at any moment. I planned to pack ten days' worth of clothes for both of us in one carry-on bag, as it was all that would fit in the back of our Lilliputian car if we brought a wheelchair. Clearly, this wasn't going to be travel as we had always known it, but we were compelled to see new places and people, history embodied in stone, and culture manifest in music and markets, and we couldn't wait to engage it all through new eyes.

We took the trip in the spring of 2012, and I had a moment of panic on the flight that—unlike every previous trip with my "pack it all in" family—Katherine and I had not really planned anything to do while in Italy. It had taken all of our attention just to plan the travel logistics. Yet there was a releasing of expectation in that moment and a relishing of precious margin and much-needed rest that we rarely gave ourselves.

Our arrival felt like we were living in *Roman Holiday*, except in a wheelchair and clown car. Nonetheless, we soaked in the sights of the gorgeous ancient hills and the quaint but terrifying alleys that I was supposed to drive through in the nearly thousand-year-old city. Thankfully, the only casualties were a few broken wheelchair spokes from pushing along the uneven stone streets of Rome, but even getting on the subway required me to help Katherine down the steep stairs with one hand while holding her folded wheelchair in my other hand. I guess accessibility for those with disabilities was not at the forefront of the Italians' consciousness—too much "la dolce vita" going on, I guess—but we made it work.

We got lost in the rolling countryside visiting local agriturismos—inns where the most amazing meals, farmed on the land, were matter-of-factly laid out on tables under pergolas covered in ancient, twisting vines, teeming with flowers overlooking lush green valleys. It was heaven. And without guilt, we spent a good amount of time in the apartment friends had offered to us, a seven-hundred-year-old structure that was once part of the church next door. Katherine sat by the wood-burning stone fireplace while I cooked food from the local market, and we talked for hours, threw log after log on the fire, napped, and cooked some more.

I turned thirty on Palm Sunday, and we attended the service at the Vatican. We had naturally arrived a bit late—on "wheelchair time," as we'd come to know it. We were strangely but warmly engaged by a series of pantalooned Vatican guards and then nun after nun, who pointed us to a path through the crowd of the thousands who had arrived earlier. As we wound our way to some unknown destination, quite certain we'd be arrested for accidentally stumbling into the pope's private quarters, we turned a final corner and saw that the path on which we had been directed led to the very front row, with only steps between us and the podium from which the pope would give the morning's message. It was jaw-dropping to be so close, but even more so to see that the entire front row was comprised of wheelchairs. We took our place in the line with "our people," and we both began to weep at the beauty of this picture. The trip had been so life-giving, but it had also been stressful and challenging to navigate, especially with the wheelchair. Yet now we were reminded that in the kingdom of God, there was a paradoxical experience of the last being first, the weak being empowered, the invisible being seen. And it was one of the most stunning pictures we had ever witnessed, like a curtain being pulled back for a moment to offer a glimpse of a different world—a world that awaited us—and it was glorious.

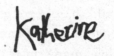

The year 2012 was joyously carefree for the Wolf family. We felt we were on an extended vacation, with an adorable four-year-old in tow. There were no major surgeries coming up, nor was I engaged in the drudgery of full-time rehab anymore. In fact, a renowned LA-based Pilates instructor, Risa Sheppard, happened to hear of my story, and knowing how much Pilates had helped her recover after her own brain injury, she offered to personally train me for free! Also, quite providentially, we were connected to Nicole Johnson, a fabulous author and dramatist, who added us to her amazing speaking team for four upcoming

"Seasons Weekend" retreats. We couldn't believe how God was opening up such incredible opportunities. We felt healthy and empowered and so excited about our future.

Jay's middle sister's wedding was scheduled for the end of June, and all three of us were in her wedding party. I was doing well enough to *walk* down the aisle with Jay on one arm and a cane in the other! I could be a bridesmaid, while James was the precious ring bearer and Jay was a groomsman. The wedding signified life moving on, post-stroke.

After the wedding, we spent more time enjoying those hot summer days in the South and treasuring being with our families in Georgia and Alabama. We took a trip to the beach with Jay's family immediately following the wedding and then tacked on an overnight trip with my dad's extended family in the mountains of South Carolina. There was an almost audible, deep sigh of *finally*. We could travel and see family and vacation and celebrate and live normally again. *We were back.*

We returned to my childhood home in Athens, where we would spend a few more days before flying out to speak at our first "official" gig for Seasons Weekend. As we were working on the messages we would share, I got up to get James a snack. The next few moments are a blur. I can remember hitting the ground, just as I had done many times before, but now, to my horror, I saw my right leg bone protruding unnaturally under the skin at mid-shin.

This was my *bad* leg. I had been working in physical therapy for almost four years to learn to put weight on this leg to teach it how to walk again. Many of my issues with walking had to do with my inability to correctly use my right leg.

As I lay on the floor of my parents' basement and waited while my mom and Jay called 911 and tried to make me more comfortable, I (thankfully) went into shock and felt no pain from the break. James came running into the hallway, announcing that he would get a Band-Aid to make it better. My maternal grandmother cried as the ambulance loaded me onto a stiff stretcher. Little did I know that I was seeing her with a fully intact mind for the final time. The woman who was among my dearest and truest friends in all the world was never the same after that day, as though something snapped in her brain as my leg snapped. Her Alzheimer's disease eerily coincided with my stroke, adding layers of sadness to our ordeal.

My parents were amazing throughout that day. My mom took care of James after we left in the ambulance. My dad came directly to the hospital with comfort (soul) food for Jay and me. Jay was the ultimate master in crisis, and he'd had plenty of practice! I knew he would deal with the EMTs and doctors and determine what should happen next.

Because of the severity of the spiral break, the team of doctors recommended the installation of a steel rod through the entire right tibia bone to form my broken leg into a functional leg again and to enable the bone to regrow correctly. Since I was stabilized, surgery was scheduled for the next morning. Those fourteen hours of waiting with a broken leg were some of the most nightmarish of my life. And Jay, yet again, found himself spending the night beside my hospital bed, sweetly complying with my delirious pleas to rub my throbbing broken leg and then to get me late-night waffles. His presence, calm and reassuring in the midst of this unexpected hell, reminded me that we had gotten through much worse, and we would get through this too.

The surgery was successful, but now I was supposed to spend a minimum of three months trying not to put any weight on my leg at all as the bone healed. I knew this terrible setback in my recovery meant that my explosive, take-no-prisoners progression toward physical restoration had come to a screeching halt, and I found that this wounding of my spirit ached worse than the pain of my broken limb.

But before long, we had a rather surprising revelation.

Because of my inability to walk after the stroke, my right leg had become pre-osteoporotic (at age thirty, no less!), which is why the bone broke so easily and so badly, thus requiring the surgeon to insert an eighteen-inch steel rod to hold it together. The rod would now be a permanent part of my "bad" right leg. In other words, while never in a million years would I have signed up for yet another surgical procedure, my weaker right leg was now reinforced with steel. Sometimes the worst thing can actually be the best thing. I was nicknamed "the Steel Magnolia" that day. I'm keeping that name for life.

I spent three weeks on a hospital bed in my parents' living room. I missed the big speaking engagement weekend in California, though I did Skype in while on heavy pain meds, which was unique to say the least. Jay slept on the living room couch next to me, giving me blood-thinner injections, tracking my medication schedule, and slowly helping me to the bedside toilet in the middle of the night. We learned a new one-legged version of the "help-me-walk dance" we had been doing since the stroke, and it was a doozy! We were eventually able to make the trip back to California and a now-different-yet-the-same life. Thankfully, we had an army behind us from all over the country. Friends from Athens and then Los Angeles brought meals for us and checked on us constantly. We continued in the sad, all-too-familiar routine of patient and caregiver, and yet there was a positive pressure to choose joy as we went through the fire yet again. Sharing our story publicly had the side benefit of encouraging us to rise to the occasion yet again, not just for ourselves, but also for those who wondered how they too might make it through their own "life breaks."

James began kindergarten that fall. It had been my goal in physical therapy all along to take him to school one day. I knew I would not be driving him, but when we bought a house less than a block from the school, I had hoped I would be a "normal mommy" who could *walk* my son to school. Now my dreams were shattered, and that loss hit me deeper than I imagined it would. It was like another dream had died—and with it some of my ability to dream into the future. Yet I was determined to see my child start this new chapter of his life, even if I had to get carried on a stretcher! Thankfully, only my wheelchair was needed, and James certainly didn't mind that I had not walked him to school. He was just happy I was there at all.

James loved going to "big boy" school, and Jay and I began to volunteer in his classroom and serve on panels and councils. When I was in James's classroom and recess time came, the kids lined up for rides in the wheelchair. Several of them asked why I was in a wheelchair, and in a way it was nice (and a relief) to have kids see my boot and assume I was wheelchair-bound solely because of my broken leg. I didn't want James to be negatively affected among his peers by my disability. As much as I understood how great it was for James to appreciate the differences in people and to stand up for the weak, I was so afraid he would be taunted because of me. Now I found that his classmates thought it was fun and even "cool" to get to ride around the playground. *Could this be happening? The wheelchair was cool to my son's new peer group?*

I was additionally blessed by the fact that the school had a children's special needs program, the only one in the district, so seeing wheelchairs was actually quite commonplace. More than that, the culture of the school was one of inclusion and concern toward those with disabilities. This was like a God wink to our little family. As we dropped off and picked up James each day, I would encounter several children at my eye level who were using my mode of transportation. I always introduced myself to them and then promptly introduced James in hopes that these kids would start being James's buddies whenever they saw each other throughout the day. Our prayer was for James to cultivate deep compassion as he learned about the world through the lens of a mommy with disabilities. Instead of being intimidated by the kids in wheelchairs who were watching the able-bodied kids at recess, we longed for James to run up to those kids and play with them.

Whenever Jay wheeled me over to the school to retrieve our little guy after a full day, my heartbeat would quicken as we rounded the corner to his classroom. Every time our "big kid" saw us, he'd let out a loud "Mom, Dad!" and would run to us. Then, since he was tired—or, as I liked to assume, since he just loved being my baby—he would climb into my lap, and Daddy would push us home.

Yes, the wheelchair was quite "cool" indeed.

Jay

The winter months following Katherine's leg break were a time of putting things to bed, a time of saying good-bye. It was a season of making peace with the need to let go of certain things in our lives, things we had loved.

As James started school that fall, it only seemed natural that he would transition to a "big kid" bed. At five years old, he was still sleeping in his original baby crib, though we had converted it into a toddler daybed. Getting a new bed was on our to-do list, but not a very high priority. Out of the blue, our dear friends Anna and Andy (the same couple who kept James for months after the stroke) offered an extra twin bed frame they were getting rid of. Andy even came over and helped me quickly disassemble the crib and set up the new bed. I posted pictures of the crib online and sold it the next day.

A few hours after we set up the bed, I rounded the corner into James's room and felt like I'd nearly had the breath knocked out of me. The room looked completely different. All of a sudden, it hit me: The crib was gone, and with it, in a way, our baby was gone too.

Around the same time, Katherine finally upgraded her well-loved cell phone to an iPhone. Her friend had taken her to the store and helped her set up the new system. I called her to check in, and it went to voice mail. I expected to hear the long-standing greeting of the Katherine from 2007, before the stroke. We had never had the heart to change it. It had become a comforting memorial of sorts, a reminder of a different Katherine with a different voice in a different life. But that day, to my surprise, I didn't hear Katherine's old voice on the greeting. Instead I heard James's voice say, "This is my mom's phone. Leave a message."

When Katherine arrived home, I felt a little stupid for being upset, but I asked her why she hadn't saved the old greeting. She replied in an earnest tone, "My voice doesn't sound like that anymore, so I decided it was time to move on." For a moment I was deeply pained at the thought of letting go of this seemingly mundane but priceless recording, this auditory snapshot from an old life erased forever. Maybe all the more so, because after four years, I found myself not being able to easily remember the sound of Katherine's original voice.

I swallowed the lump in my throat and resolved that she was right. After all, fully embracing a new life would be impossible without letting go of some of the remnants of our old life, even dearly loved ones.

One night, out of the blue, James told me, "Dad, I don't like hearts."

"Why, James?" I asked confusedly.

"Because hearts break," he said matter-of-factly.

As a parent, those are the moments that sting the most, when you know your child has glimpsed the reality of this world a bit sooner than you would have liked. Nonetheless, James and C. S. Lewis had it right: "To love at all is to be vulnerable.

Love anything, and your heart will be wrung and possibly be broken."* If the alternative to a broken heart is an "unbreakable, impenetrable, irredeemable" one, as Lewis suggested, then I suppose the choice is clear. But for any of us, when our heart has been broken as the result of loving something, we can't help but question if the love was worth the pain.

Katherine and I knelt beside James's big boy bed that night and said our nightly prayers for him, over him. It was perhaps the one constant in his rather nontraditional upbringing. And we always sang the song I had sung when I asked Katherine to marry me, the blessing that was not right but perfect still. The song reminded us of our blessings, not because we were perfect, but because our heavenly Father was.

James closed his eyes and smiled contentedly. He had grown from a baby into a boy, and it was wondrous to look at his face as various images of the baby born before life changed flashed before me and were superimposed on top of him. His eyes, the same now as when he was new, had seen more than most his age, but we prayed that all he had seen would inform all he would do. As Katherine prayed over her son in her new voice that was rich with joy and sorrow, I knew that the loving, even with the losing, was all worth it.

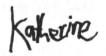

We had been telling this unfolding story of our lives for nearly five years, and we viewed our roles not just as authors or protagonists but also as stewards. Speaking and blogging were our main forms of communicating, but there were limitations. We had stayed in Los Angeles after the stroke at least in part

---

* C. S. Lewis, *The Four Loves* (New York: Harcourt, Brace, 1960), 121.

because of its role in telling stories to the culture at large. It seemed to be the appropriate time to leverage our connections in this city so we might tell our story through one of the most powerful mediums of all—film.

A friend of ours from church, D.J. Viola, was a working director with an impressive résumé, but more than that, he had been in Jay's men's group and had thoughtfully considered our story for years, asking us some of the more insightful questions of anyone in our lives. We knew we needed a creative and objective voice to help us see the big picture and the important themes of this complex series of moments and emotions. How in the world could we cram years of struggle into a short, engaging video?

After much discussion with D.J., we pulled the trigger and began to schedule the shoot and assemble the crew. Rather than squeezing free favors out of everyone, we felt compelled to pay them all something for their troubles. Appropriately, we raised funds from our digital audience, and in the end, we raised double the amount of our proposed budget, which encouraged us deeply, assuring us that our story was one that people, strangers even, wanted us to keep telling. It was so meaningful to have the very community that had long engaged our story online be the one to help create this more tangible representation of it—one that would be shared with even more people online.

The film turned out beautifully. Parts of it made us smile, while other parts made us weep every time we watched it. We premiered the film to our friends at our annual joint birthday party, which by then was deemed a "Happy Everything" celebration since it was also close to my stroke survival anniversary.

The huge response to the film and the process of seeing our story come to life cinematically inspired us to take one of the biggest leaps of faith in our adult lives—working together in full-time ministry. We had been ministering online and in person "on the side" for many years, ever since the stroke, really.

We squeezed in speaking and writing and connecting with fellow sufferers between therapy and legal consultant work and parenthood. While it had clearly been fruitful, we knew we had been given a unique opportunity, one that would greatly benefit from both of us focusing on it full-time. Though it was daunting to think of working together from home on a start-up ministry, we had seen God's provision in everything He had called us to, and we wanted to be faithful. We jumped in.

Using his hard-earned legal skills, Jay put together the beastly 501(c)(3) nonprofit application and organized the business side of this new operation. Jay's youngest sister, Alex, tirelessly offered her time and expertise in creating a new website and doing all the graphic design elements. Though separated by ten years and thousands of miles, they grew closer as adult friends in their creative collaboration.

It was exciting to transition into these new, more official roles, and it was humbling to recognize that this great calling on our lives was born out of the greatest tragedy of our lives. As opportunities and financial support, prayers, and clarity came pouring in, we knew we had made the right decision. God was making something new out of our story, and in the process He was making something new out of us as well.

Just before school started up for James in the late summer of 2013, we crawled into bed early one night. It had been a full few weeks since Katherine had the painful screws from her broken leg surgery removed, and we had just returned from a wonderful weekend of ministry and reuniting with old friends. We were tired in the best way, and sleep came easily as the fan softly whirred overhead.

My next conscious moment came in disjointed flashes as my brain frantically tried to contextualize dreams with reality, sound with sight. I don't remember even turning on the light or getting out of bed—just standing above Katherine as she lay facedown in the corner of our bedroom, legs splayed out unnaturally, wrapped in our bedsheets, her head jammed between the bedside table and the wall.

I gingerly wrapped my arms around her torso and carefully lifted her up. As I turned her toward me, I saw that her face was covered in blood. My measured tone belied my quivering nerves as I surmised that the source of the blood seemed to be her "good" eye. I helped her up and calmed her. Then I quickly ascertained that the wound was on her eyebrow bone, not in her eye. *Thank You, Lord!* But when the gash opened and I could see the bone like a ravine through her flesh, I briskly walked to the bathroom, as I felt I might pass out. I splashed some cold water on my face, took a few deep breaths, and then jumped back into the bloody fray, bringing ice and towels and a single Band-Aid, which was almost comical.

Katherine began to weep at the thought of waking James and shuttling him to our neighbor's house for an impromptu sleepover. The ripple effects of her medical issues on our family were always deeply troubling to her. I somehow convinced her to come with me to the ER, as James would actually love the midnight, bed-swapping adventure, and my subpar sewing and stitching skills were likely to give her a Spock-like, permanently raised eyebrow.

We made it to UCLA's ER in no time at that late hour, quickly traversing the usually busy interstate. Going to this particular place might make a normal person's pulse quicken and stomach flutter, but for us, going to a hospital felt strangely like going home. It was a place where we had found safety and help over the course of many years. We had been to a dozen different specialists at UCLA, so the place had a comforting quality for us.

And if the worst thing happened, as it had at points in the past, we knew we would be well taken care of there.

The waiting room was dimly lit and quiet, save for a few disheveled inhabitants. Surprisingly we made it to an examination room within a half hour. When the on-call doctor arrived, I took the lead, explaining Katherine's history and what I ascertained had happened. My perceived forcefulness, as well as an ill-timed joke from Katherine about me pushing her out of bed, resulted in the doctor asking me to step outside of the room.

For a moment, I felt slapped in the face. I was the one who got woken up from a dead sleep for an ER visit, and now the insinuation was that I might be to blame! I realized that such precautions are founded in real threats and that even people who are innocent must be subjected to the same scrutiny as those who are guilty, all for the greater good. My heart suddenly broke for those women forcibly brought to that same ER by men who didn't feel the same unstoppable goodwill for them that I felt for my wife.

When I reentered the exam room, Katherine was engaged in conversation with the nurse and doctor, both of whom were amazed at her post-stroke recovery. These were opportunities our story gave us to personify intangible hope in flesh and bone. We gave our Hope Heals cards to these new hearers and directed them on how to find our short film.

"I might cry," the nurse lamented.

"Maybe," Katherine said. "But wait for the end. It's the best part—the hopeful part."

As they began stitching back together the broken place, I instinctively turned on our iPod and began rubbing Katherine's feet to distract her. A song called "Beautiful Things" by a Christian husband-and-wife band, Gungor, came on.

Katherine told the doctor, "We're Christians, in case you couldn't tell by the music. Is it okay if we play this?"

The doctor replied, "As long as it's not hate-filled—of course you may. I want you to be comfortable."

The lyrics warmed the cold room, speaking of hope and beauty birthed from chaos and dust. It was a welcome distraction and a reminder that broken places were being mended all around. The song ended, and the doctor whispered, "That was beautiful."

After Katherine's eyebrow was redefined with a row of stitches spanning nearly its full length, we drove home around 3:00 a.m. on the even quieter interstate. We pulled through an all-night drive-thru for an ice cream cone to share. When we settled back into bed, sleep did not come as easily as it had much earlier that night. I wrapped my arm over Katherine with a steely, seat belt-like resolve—not the most comfortable position but perhaps the most comforting for us both.

We knew all too well that no single one of us knows what tomorrow holds or even what the night holds, for that matter. It is unnatural, against every animal instinct in us, to release ourselves into that reality; but God calls us there—to that place of surrender where He invites us to rest, secure in arms more capable and more loving than our own.

That night was not our last hospital visit, nor was it the last time we fell asleep holding each other tightly. That late-night visit to the ER challenged us to sit with the question of suffering and to consider it deeply. As our ministry and connections to more hurting people grew, we continued to find that sacrifice is the central theme of love and faith, and we asked ourselves how they all connected. What if the good resulting from our pain inured not to our own benefit but to the benefit of strangers?

We were seeing humanity with different eyes as we recognized that we were being asked to sacrifice things we held dear so that someone else, perhaps someone we would never know, might find the hope they needed. Were we willing to lie down on altars or hospital beds, enduring all manner of loss, so that something truly lost might be found, so that a prodigal might become a beloved child? It became clearer and clearer that this was our calling—to play our role in divine appointments, to be vessels overflowing with hope for a good greater than just our own.

Katherine

In the early fall of 2013, I had my annual MRI to check the status of my brain aneurysm. We enlisted our community to pray that the aneurysm had not grown. Some had even fervently prayed there would be no sign of the aneurysm at all. We also had asked for the past three years for God to miraculously remove it from my brain. Sadly, the latest scans indicated it was still there, though it had not grown. The prospect of a future of scans and waiting on the results gave me a sick feeling in the pit of my stomach. We talked and talked about this aneurysm with Dr. Gonzales, who clearly did not want me to have to undergo another brain surgery, but it was becoming more evident that this time bomb needed to be removed.

There were three factors that informed our decision to go ahead with the operation. The first was that if the aneurysm would ever rupture, there was an instant fatality rate of 50 percent. Though there was not a high probability of rupture at that time, I had already experienced one of those "probably won't ever happen to me" types of medical situations. That reality made it almost unthinkable to not get it removed.

The second reason to operate was our desire to grow our family. A safe pregnancy would not be possible if I had an aneurysm. Because body fluid greatly increases during pregnancy, the aneurysm could grow in size and even rupture as a result. At the age of thirty-one, I felt it would be tragic to have no option to have more biological children because of another brain issue.

Third, I asked Dr. Gonzales what he would do if I was his daughter. He looked at me with tears in his eyes and said, "I would operate. You are like a daughter to me." After that, the choice was clear.

Surgery was scheduled for the end of November, just before Thanksgiving. Obviously, this was totally different from the instantaneous nature of the first brain surgery. This time I had months to think and "prepare" (obsess) over the worst-case scenarios. While aneurysm rupture and death during surgery were rare, the possibility remained. I tried not to think about the surgery as it hung over my head throughout the fall. I kept busy during the day; however, early in the morning and late at night, my fears would often torment me.

On Sunday morning, the day before the surgery, I woke up at 4:00 a.m. in quite a state. I started crying and thinking through what would happen the next day. I decided to grab my phone and type out my will for Jay to read in case I died in surgery. As I typed, I decided to also write a letter to him. I asked him to please remarry. I told him to move where we'd always wanted to grow old together. I told him that James needed a mother and I wanted a woman in their lives. I typed that I knew we had begun Hope Heals so a widower would have a ministry of hope to heal his broken heart. By now, it was 4:30 a.m., and I was sobbing so loudly that Jay woke up and tried to console me. I reluctantly put my phone away and tried to go back to sleep.

Before I could, my phone buzzed, alerting me to an email. It was a forwarded message from a sweet friend in Alabama who was having her morning quiet time. She had received pastor John Piper's e-devotional, and the message for that day was from Hebrews 6:19: "We have this hope as an anchor for the soul, firm and secure." Jay and I love this verse—our ministry is based on it! I read the devotional and then clicked to watch a related sermon on the topic.

After watching the sermon in full, I put aside any further thoughts of will writing. It was not as if I had never heard any teaching on that powerful Scripture, but I needed to revisit the truths I already knew in order to deal with my crippling anxiety. Sometimes the most familiar truths can unexpectedly be the most powerful ones in our lives.

Sweet friends had planned a prayer time for us between the morning services at church that day. Jay, James, and I were seated in the middle of a circle, with more than a hundred people laying hands on us and spontaneously praying out loud. We all wept. The words and truth spoken over me were sweet salve to my battered soul. Engaging the body of Christ was the best decision we made that morning, though we could just as easily have chosen to isolate ourselves at home. We knew we were experiencing the beauty of Galatians 6:2: "Carry each other's burdens, and in this way you will fulfill the law of Christ."

After leaving church, Jay had planned a special trip to the Getty Museum. The Getty is one of our favorite spots in all of Los Angeles, full of memories for us and overflowing with great beauty—an often overlooked attribute that is vital to engage when pain, fear, and death abound. True beauty viscerally connects us to God and reminds us, in ways platitudes cannot, that we are beautiful to Him.

We lay on a blanket spread across the lawn of the museum garden after eating a delicious lunch. If this, for some reason, were to be my last afternoon with my guys, I could not think of a better way to spend it. By nightfall, I was calm. I felt a special kind of Christian peace that doesn't quite make sense in a way I don't think I had ever felt before. I was ready for the surgery that I knew in my soul would lead me right into what God had next for my life.

The operation went just as planned. A catheter was delicately threaded from the femoral artery in my thigh all the way to the carotid artery in my brain, where it filled my aneurysm full of microscopic platinum coils, all expertly guided by the hand of my friend Dr. Gonzalez. Placing this foreign object into my brain caused weeks of the most intense headaches of my life. This was part of the process of healing. And the healing hurt, as it always does.

That Thanksgiving, my family gathered around our dining room table as they had gathered in the waiting room just days before. It was hard not to recall my first Thanksgiving after the stroke five years before, the one when I could not eat or do anything, but when I also began to truly know that God Himself was enough. And we gave thanks for it all. It seemed that these cycles of hardship and thanksgiving and celebration and joy and loss and hope were not singular, disconnected events, but rather a cycle that would continue throughout my life. It was this very cycle that would inspire me to continue to truly live.

It had been nearly a year since Katherine's aneurysm surgery. It seemed we were living in the afterglow of yet another second chance at life, which enlivened us to get back into the world in ways we had not since the stroke. "Hope Heals" bloomed as we traveled and spoke and sought to love hurting people well. Yet now, we found ourselves once again sitting in the white-walled exam room for Katherine's annual neuro appointment. Some of our visits to Dr. Gonzalez over the past several years had been almost giddy with relief, while others had shockingly kicked us in the gut. Those visits were reminders that, by all accounts, Katherine should not be here.

The exam room became a place of quiet reflection for us both as we contemplated the long journey following Katherine's near-death and resurrection of sorts. We were grateful beyond words that she had lived, yet we couldn't help but remember what had died along the way. In so many places, the flesh of our stories had been wounded, both figuratively and literally, creating lines of demarcation between a life that is and one that will never be. If we expected time to heal all our wounds, then what were we to do with the scars that remained?

When Jesus appeared to His disciples after the resurrection, His body still bore the scars that had saved us all. Perhaps His scars will be the only ones in heaven, but I wondered if our own scars, both external and internal, will be on full display too as holy reminders of the wounds we suffered on the way home.

The door to the exam room cracked open, and we looked up expectantly at Dr. Gonzalez. This time, blessedly, he had a smile on his face. "The aneurysm site looks wonderful; it's scarred over, almost as if it had never been there at all. And the place where we removed the AVM shows no signs of residual malformation."

We embraced our friend, our eyes wet and our throats tight. This was the outcome we had long desired, though one we weren't sure we would ever get. In a sense, Katherine's brain was finally healed.

One day, we will see. One day, the arc of our stories will all make perfect sense. One day, we will trace the lines of our scars and find them to have fallen in the most pleasant of places, to see in them our great inheritance. One day, we won't need to hope, nor will we need to be healed because we will be face-to-face with the source of both, the source of everything . . . Jesus.

And in the glory of His face, the darkest suffering and loss we have endured will fade like shadows at daybreak. Until then, the moments of releasing our lives into the hands of a God we cannot see are the closest to wholeness we will come on this side of eternity. This is our truest healing—the healing of our souls—and it sustains us when we wake up tomorrow to an unknown but hopeful new day.

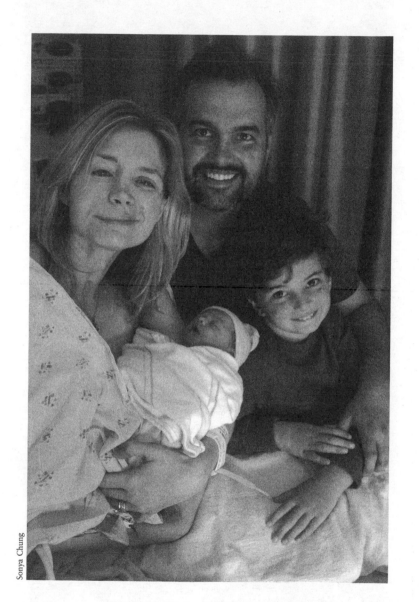

Sonya Chung

EPILOGUE

Katherine

The state of California deemed me permanently disabled in the fall of 2010. As a twenty-eight-year-old woman, I was enrolled in Medicare; my driver's license was revoked; and I was issued a permanent handicapped license plate for our car. Since the stroke, I've had eleven surgeries, and I will likely have to have more, maybe many more, in the future. I still don't walk well or use my right hand well, and I don't eat, speak, see, or hear normally either. I currently have both osteoporosis and arthritis. This thirty-three-year-old body feels more like that of an eighty-three-year-old. This has been a difficult assignment, to say the least.

However, over the past seven years of this saga, I have learned to do many things well—to wait well, suffer well, cope well, persevere well, and even to lose well. Our culture tells us to succeed, be beautiful, avoid pain, and be happy. What if everything important in our lives is actually the opposite?

Maybe it takes life being *undeniably* terrible before we can *truly* recognize *its undeniable splendor.*

Suffering powerfully informs who I am now. While awful and painful, affliction has led to a heartbreaking but beautiful deepening in me. I have learned to embrace the suffering. I have learned to not push back, but to lean in hard when it hurts the most and press on. Pain has been an instructor, teaching me deeper truths about myself and God and bringing me closer to Christ in a way I never was before this happened. The pain has weighed heavily on our shoulders and hearts, threatening to crush us, but we have not been crushed. The hope in our hearts has always been greater than despair because it anchors us.

Our hope is Jesus. We trust Him and all He is doing—in all that we understand and, more importantly, in all that we do not.

I believe we are all here for purposes beyond ourselves and beyond our comprehension. We were born to know and to manifest the God who heals our souls and calls us into the kind of life that doesn't end with death.

Two weeks after our appointment with Dr. Gonzalez, which confirmed the healing of my brain, we returned to Hawaii, the place where we honeymooned, to celebrate our tenth wedding anniversary. Those first ten years of marriage weren't ones we would ever have chosen for ourselves or our child. Yet we remembered them, celebrated them, and even gave thanks for them, knowing, quite surprisingly, that we would not change them because if we removed the depth of our sufferings, we would also remove the power of our hope. Those ten years were the precedent not just of pain but of purpose—and they will inform the next ten years and the next after that.

While we were on Kauai, Jay opened the fridge in our friend's condo one day, and I experienced something I hadn't in a long time: The smell of leftover pizza was disgustingly intense. I knew right then . . . I was pregnant. It was the earliest kind of pregnancy test from a person who has developed an acute awareness of her body. Getting pregnant just two weeks after effectively getting the go-ahead from Dr. Gonzalez was perhaps the only medical "shortcut" in my life so far.

⚓

I had longed for another child for nearly seven years. Even a few months after my stroke, I tried to convince Jay that we should get pregnant. After all, we were already in the hospital! It made total sense to my clouded brain. Yet I think my longing for a baby reflected the most visceral longing we all have—for new life to be born in us. Years later, as I wrote this book, looking down at my pregnant belly pulsing with a baby we never thought would be, the beauty of the gospel had never been more vibrant: near death into newness of life.

On June 26, 2015, John Nestor Wolf came into this world two weeks early but perfectly on time. Our prayers for a noneventful C-section were answered in a spectacularly ordinary fashion, as John came so quickly and so effortlessly, without even a push, that there was no time for an epidural, let alone another surgery. John was born in the triage room. They even had to rush in a birthing table attachment at the last second. And just over my shoulder, out that room's window, we could see the old hospital building, the place where my life was saved and regained seven years before. We both wept at all the ways in which our invisible God makes Himself as plain as day, so we might remember, so we might not be afraid. John was born at 7:07 a.m. The number seven often represents completion, and it seemed clear that one season was finished and a new one had begun.

The name John means "the Lord has been gracious." In the Bible, there are two men named John who were integral to the life and ministry of Jesus. The first, John the Baptist, "came as a witness to testify concerning that light . . . the true light that gives light to everyone" (John 1:7, 9). The second, John the apostle (brother of James, no less)—"the disciple whom Jesus loved" (John 13:23)—told of a man who was born blind "so that the works of God might be displayed in him" (John 9:3).

John's middle name, Nestor, honors Dr. Nestor Gonzalez, whose life's work has been giving second chances to patients like me. The name Nestor means "wisdom," "remembrance," "homecoming," and "seeker of miracles." And whenever someone asks the origin of John's nontraditional middle name, he'll have a chance to tell this story.

And in the telling of his story, like all our stories, he will bear witness to light in the darkness and life out of death, to a God who saved his mommy and in so doing saved him too.

ACKNOWLEDGMENTS

Years ago, while still in brain rehab, I excitedly told my therapist we wanted to write a book. She lovingly responded, "Everyone says that. They all want to make sense of their pain and share it to help others, but the reality of life after a stroke rarely allows for luxuries like book writing." And yet she left us with this charge: "But you be the ones to do it."

In the midst of disabilities and distractions, new normals and unknown futures, we remembered her motivating words, and we did it. We wrote this book to tell our story, but also to tell the stories of those who cannot tell their own.

To our families, we most certainly could not have stewarded our story were it not for your love so graciously lavished on us. Without your tireless support, physical presence, and constant affirmations, we would never have been unleashed to minister and share our story, let alone write a book. We love you and thank you all for giving us the great gift of being able to witness the coming full circle of our tragedy into redemption.

To our Los Angeles community, specifically our church family at Bel Air Presbyterian and our small group, you have shown us what it means to enter into and carry each other's burdens and have given us a beautiful glimpse of the kingdom of God alive and at work in the world. You've breathed life and hope into so many dead places in our hearts. You've stunningly made our intangible God tangible when we needed Him the most.

To our digital community, made up of so many of our

hometown cheerleaders from Athens, Georgia, and Montgomery, Alabama, we thank you for spurring us on to tell our story and to live out a better story in the process. Your longtime prayers, financial support, and unstoppable goodwill have reminded us that we are never alone. You have changed the outcomes of our lives and, in so doing, changed the outcomes of the lives of those whom our story has and will touch.

To our team at Zondervan and Alive, we are humbled by the opportunity to partner with you to share the story of our great pain and our great purpose. To Carolyn McCready and Traci Mullins, thank you for taking our words and making them shine, all the while speaking encouragement and truth into our insecurities and fears. To Lisa Jackson, thank you for seeing us as worthy storytellers and guiding us in this new world. To our friend Nicole Johnson and the Seasons Weekend team, we would not be writing this book were it not for you, quite literally connecting us to Carolyn, but even more, you have given us the unique and empowering gift of trusting us to tell our story and of nurturing the good things you see in us—things we didn't even see in ourselves.

To our medical team, which continues to grow and grow, specifically the world-renowned UCLA Medical Center and Casa Colina Hospital and Centers for Healthcare, you helped save my life but also equipped me to live the new life that remains and, in so doing, to take the comfort we have received and give it to those in need. From the doctors and nurses to the therapists and techs, from the social workers and the janitors to the volunteers, administrators, and trustees, thank you for living into your unique calling to help patients and families like us. Though you may rarely see the outcomes or receive the loudest praise, your work matters. Thank you so much.

To our beloved Dr. Nestor Gonzalez, I would not be here—we would not be here—without you. Your life's work has given life to so many. Your sacrifices have not been wasted. You have planted the seeds of hope and healing, which have blossomed with profound beauty in the midst of a despairing world. God's love and compassion flow through you. We thank you, dear friend, for the gift of a second chance.

To our sons, James and John, you make our hearts flutter; you are the best medicine and a great source of inspiration; and you challenge us to know and accept the love and grace of God anew every day. We wrote this book for you, James, as a prayer of remembrance for the unexpected course your life has taken—to heal the hurts and fortify the hopes that will be uniquely yours as a result of it. We wrote this book for you, John, as a love letter to your improbable life, so you might know its miraculous beginnings and long to live out your own story of grace to the very end.

VERSES CITED
IN PART THREE

For you [LORD] created my inmost being;
    you knit me together in my mother's womb.
I praise you because I am fearfully and wonderfully made;
    your works are wonderful,
    I know that full well.
Psalm 139:13–14

Consider it pure joy, my brothers and sisters, whenever you face
trials of many kinds, because you know that the testing of your
faith produces perseverance.
James 1:2–3

And we know that in all things God works for the good of those
who love him, who have been called according to his purpose.
Romans 8:28

The LORD will fight for you; you need only to be still.
Exodus 14:14

In all my prayers for all of you, I always pray with joy . . . being
confident of this, that he who began a good work in you will
carry it on to completion until the day of Christ Jesus.
Philippians 1:4, 6

And the God of all grace, who called you to his eternal glory in Christ, after you have suffered a little while, will himself restore you and make you strong, firm and steadfast. To him be the power for ever and ever. Amen.

1 Peter 5:10–11

I remain confident of this:
    I will see the goodness of the LORD
    in the land of the living.
Wait for the LORD;
    be strong and take heart
    and wait for the LORD.

Psalm 27:13–14

As a prisoner for the Lord, then, I urge you to live a life worthy of the calling you have received.

Ephesians 4:1

Therefore we do not lose heart. Though outwardly we are wasting away, yet inwardly we are being renewed day by day. For our light and momentary troubles are achieving for us an eternal glory that far outweighs them all. So we fix our eyes not on what is seen, but on what is unseen, since what is seen is temporary, but what is unseen is eternal.

2 Corinthians 4:16–17

31901059711624